FOREIGN MEDICAL GRADUATES

IN THE UNITED STATES

FOREIGN MEDICAL GRADUATES
IN THE UNITED STATES

Harold Margulies / Lucille Stephenson Bloch

A COMMONWEALTH FUND BOOK

HARVARD UNIVERSITY PRESS   1969

Cambridge, Massachusetts

PREFACE

During the past twenty years foreign medical graduates (FMGs) have come to the United States in increasing numbers. Their education, professional activities, and migration have been a source of growing concern to responsible persons here and abroad. The records of the American Medical Association, the Association of American Medical Colleges, and the American Hospital Association, to name only a few of the organizations most directly involved, reveal an impressive list of conferences, steering committee reports, special studies, and thoughtful comments on the subject.

The issues are now more than ever before in need of both professional and public consideration. In the past few years the number of FMGs arriving annually in the United States has increased markedly, thus heightening national interest as the associated problems become more apparent. Many of the ideas being expressed today have been stated before, but there remains great uncertainty regarding the best ways to resolve these problems.

The whole subject of physician migration merits a critical review, which is the purpose of this monograph. We shall concentrate on certain specific problems which deserve special attention and thus our review will be selective rather than definitive. We have deliberately excluded from our analyses those FMGs who represent the United States' most successful educational efforts and the least frequent sources of brain drain. Throughout this century organizations like the Rockefeller Foundation and various governmental agencies such as the Agency for International Development (AID) and the Public

PREFACE

Health Service have supported FMGs who have studied in the
United States and subsequently returned to their own countries.
Many of these physicians have since become important national
and international figures in and outside the field of medicine,
and thousands more have returned to less prominent but nevertheless vital roles in their nations' health services. Regrettably,
these individuals are few in number and are virtually lost in the
present large wave of migration. Furthermore, there has been
a steady decline in support for such specifically designed activities.[1] Had all FMGs come to the United States through such
prudently planned programs the issues of the day would be
different and much less troublesome.[2]

Similarly, we shall not comment on some of the positive
aspects of FMG migration that have proved particularly beneficial to the United States. This country has received from other
countries many outstanding teachers and research scientists who
have contributed notably to our society and its institutions.
Other FMGs have been of great service to the communities in
which they practice medicine.

We have not included any full discussion of the relevance of
the FMG's training in the United States to the needs of his home
country. That subject deserves a separate study, but it is considered in our discussion of the FMG while he is in this country.

This monograph has been written for several reasons. One of
these is to present the data that are available on FMGs and to
indicate the areas where data are either nonexistent or unde-
pendable. The material on this topic has been collected over a
period of several years. Because there is so much speculation
and so much erroneous information being published on the
subject, we feel that factual information is now more than ever
necessary. There is a need for presentation of the data which are
available as well as for identification of the gaps in our knowledge where data are now unavailable. An appendix has been
included to present relevant additional and up-to-date statistics
to which reference will be made in the various chapters.

Further, this study attempts to provide a synopsis of the most influential factors that affect the migration of FMGs to the United States. While the authors do not pretend to have offered a complete study of the complex issues of migration, they feel, along with many others, that this is one of the more important questions facing the United States today. Simply stated, the liberalized immigration laws of the United States have resulted in an influx of foreign physicians from the developing areas of the world, physicians who may or may not return to their homelands but who are, in any event, filling manpower needs in this country for a considerable period of time.

As the former Assistant Secretary of State for Cultural Affairs, Charles Frankel, said: "This is one of the steady, trying, troublesome issues confronted by our government." [3] World opinion from New Delhi to Trafalgar Square has been building up constantly over the so-called "brain drain." On August 25, 1967 an international conference of ten nations convened in Lausanne, Switzerland to discuss this topic and outline possible multilateral approaches to its solution. In October 1967 the British Ministry of Health sent a team of doctors to the United States in an attempt to repatriate some of their physicians. Other nations, such as India, Canada, and Greece, to name a few, are trying various means of inducing their skilled personnel to return home. Great Britain is offering to pay the return fare for its expatriate physicians in North America. Some countries make definite commitments of positions in their recruitment efforts, while others are actively engaged in establishing contact with their physicians abroad and informing them of the possibilities in their home countries.

Meanwhile, throughout the world newspapers are reporting that India will no longer allow the examination of the Educational Council for Foreign Medical Graduates (ECFMG) to be given, or that the "Brain Drain has saved the U. S. £357 Million," or that the "Medical Brain Drain is a Tragic Loss for Korea." The Minister of Health for Israel publicly agreed with

PREFACE

the British Minister of Health's statement that he was not prepared to "invest thousands of pounds sterling in a medical student only to increase the membership of the American Medical
Association." [4]

International concern with migration is not new. What is new
is our increasing awareness of the ways in which the movements
of people alter the pace of socioeconomic development. Throughout the world there is an increasing respect for the usefulness
of talented and skilled individuals who can effectively exploit
the massive technical knowledge that dominates our civilization.
The gap between rich and poor nations is plain to see. The
economic forces of "push" and "pull" are increasingly obvious.
Although the poor will not become richer through better use of
indigenous brain power alone, without it their prospects are
very bleak indeed.[5]

The United States has assumed a heavy responsibility in its
efforts to help satisfy the ambitions of less fortunate countries
to acquire skills and knowledge comparable with our own. We
have provided unparalleled opportunities for a full range of
education and training for tens of thousands of citizens from
other countries. Medical teaching centers, large and small,
located in every part of the country have provided free access
to their educational programs for those whose opportunities at
home are limited. Physicians have come from every continent
for training in public health, for Ph.D. studies in basic medical
sciences, and for clinical and research experience. For years
academic and professional societies have pondered the ways in
which our institutions can best serve those of less developed
countries without compromising our standards of excellence or
our internal responsibilities. Selection procedures have been
reviewed and revised; medical educators have discussed common interests with their counterparts abroad; and hundreds of
physicians have participated directly in overseas educational
programs.

Our good intentions are unprecedented in world history. They have been complicated, ironically, by the concomitant relaxation of immigration policies and by the fact that the help we provide is itself a powerful advertisement for the great advantages of life in an affluent society.

In an effort to face the criticisms that have been engendered by the very fact of migration and to analyze their meaning as well as their validity, we shall focus on the migration of physicians as one of its major themes. The monograph's scope will be limited to an analysis of FMGs who have already migrated to the United States. Although patterns of migration affect many skilled individuals other than those in the health professions, there are issues unique to physicians that justify this special attention.

Physicians who migrate to the United States create a number of special problems, only some of which are readily apparent. An especially important question is whether FMGs provide medical care of high enough quality. This must be judged by standards which we believe are essential to this country's national well being. The medical education provided in the United States to achieve such standards is prohibitively expensive for most of the countries from which FMGs migrate. The issue is magnified by the growing acceptance of good health care as a basic human right and complicated by the shortages of health manpower which limit the United States' capacity to meet national needs without dependence upon resources other than our own.

In contrast with students who come to the United States for other types of training, physicians emigrate after they have become fully qualified to provide direct and urgently needed services to their people. They depart from their own countries after they have already benefited from a large investment in their knowledge, but before they have actually been of use to those who have supported them.

In further contrast with other foreign students, the graduate education which FMGs receive in our hospitals includes a major participation in direct patient care. This service to patients is provided with varying degrees of supervision, but in essence it represents a significant addition to United States health manpower resources. Our tradition of graduate medical training has encouraged a stay of five years for physicians who have come here through the Exchange Visitor program, thus increasing their contribution to our communities and, conversely, the loss to the communities they have temporarily or permanently abandoned. For these and other reasons, including marriage to American citizens, physicians have been far more successful than have others in their attempts to obtain visa waivers which will allow them to remain permanently. (Table B5 in the Appendix illustrates this point quite clearly.)

Most of the physicians and other health personnel who migrate to the United States come from developing countries, whereas the majority of other foreign students do not.[6] This increases significantly the total effect of the separation of these individuals from their own countries, particularly when it is now evident that our own manpower shortages are providing almost unlimited opportunities for the employment of foreign medical graduates. The demand for more physicians, particularly in our hospitals, has created a market for FMGs which frequently overrides all other considerations.

Finally, the migration of physicians to the United States is influenced by the fragmented series of regulatory mechanisms that govern their entry, stay, and departure. This disparate system includes governmental and nongovernmental agencies and professional bodies whose specific obligations and responsibilities are at times conflicting and as a whole lack unity. As a consequence, an understanding of physician migration requires critical appreciation of the specific character of each component of the controlling mechanisms. Similarly, sensible solutions to the issues can be devised only through revisions which produce order and consistency within a democratic framework and without the loss of what has already proved satisfactory.

Another basic objective of this monograph is to analyze the impact of FMGs on medicine in the United States. With FMGs becoming an increasingly meaningful factor in our health manpower, it is only logical to study their characteristics and their contributions. Too little has been done in this area, although much has been said. Some information, such as that dealing with the professional activities of FMGs, their major sources of income, their areas of specialization, and their performance on licensing examinations, is available and included in this monograph. Also, several special studies of certain areas of FMG activities have been made and will be commented upon.

Finally, this study, after defining and presenting the FMG in the United States setting, seeks to make some suggestions for the resolution of the problem which the FMG presents, one which has often been discussed but without appropriate efforts to find solutions.

There have been years in which to study the impact of foreign physicians on American medicine, but the problem has continued to grow and to expand until today the brain drain question has pushed the FMGs into prominence once more. By bringing together all of the diverse elements involved in the FMG subject, this monograph will attempt to offer some guidelines for changes in the present situation, changes which may serve the best interests of all nations by providing appropriate devices for continuing improvements in the ensuing years.

The authors are indebted to many people for their assistance and advice during the preparation of this monograph. To list them all would be an exhaustive exercise, and we feel certain that those most intimately involved with this subject will recognize their contributions quite readily without being named.

There are some who deserve a special word of thanks, for

without their cooperation, the writing of this monograph would have been manifestly more difficult. In particular, the authors would like to express their deep appreciation to the Association of American Medical Colleges, the Agency for International Development, and the National Advisory Commission on Health Manpower, under whose support and auspices this project was conceived and through which most of the background work was accomplished. The authors are indebted to Henry van Zile Hyde, M.D., Director of the Division of International Medical Education of the AAMC, for his encouragement of this monograph.

Many of the statistics presented here were obtained through the cooperation of the American Medical Association, the Immigration and Naturalization Service, the Educational Council for Foreign Medical Graduates, the United Nations, the Association of American Medical Colleges, and the U.S. Department of State. Each of these organizations was helpful at all times, although they are not responsible for any interpretations of the statistical material which they supplied.

All of the opinions and interpretations which are expressed in this monograph are those of the authors and are not the responsibility of the individuals or organizations which assisted with the study.

From time to time throughout this monograph the authors have critically reviewed and analyzed certain conditions prevailing in the United States today. At all times we have endeavored to remain objective in our interpretation of the facts. Nevertheless, we are aware of the probability that some may disagree with our conclusions. Our hope is to stimulate thinking on this subject and to encourage constructive, thoughtful solutions to a most difficult and complex issue.

Harold Margulies, M.D.
Lucille Stephenson Bloch
October 1968

CONTENTS

TABLES

CHARTS

ABBREVIATIONS AND GLOSSARY

AAMC	Association of American Medical Colleges
AHA	American Hospital Association
AMA	American Medical Association
Bull. N.Y. Acad. Med.	*Bulletin of the New York Academy of Medicine*
ECFMG	Educational Council for Foreign Medical Graduates
FMG	Foreign Medical Graduate
INS	Immigration and Naturalization Service
JAMA	*Journal of the American Medical Association*
J. Med. Educ.	*Journal of Medical Education*
New Engl. J. Med.	*New England Journal of Medicine*
PAHO	Pan American Health Organization
USMG	United States or Canadian Medical Graduate
WHO	World Health Organization

ACCREDITED HOSPITAL: A United States hospital which is certified by the Joint Commission on Accreditation of Hospitals (The American Medical Association, the American Hospital Association, the American College of Physicians, and the American College of Surgeons make up the Joint Commission).

AFFILIATED HOSPITAL: A United States hospital which is associated with a medical school and uses that hospital for teaching purposes.

DSP/66 FORM: A certificate which the Department of State gives to hospitals with approved internship and residency programs for issuance to foreign medical graduates who qualify for Exchange Visitor status.

EXCHANGE VISITOR: Any person qualifying to visit the United States as a student, teacher, trainee, or leader under the provisions of the "Mutual Educational and Cultural Exchange Act of 1961."

HOSPITAL WITH APPROVED INTERNSHIPS AND RESIDENCIES: A United States hospital which has one or more of its internship and residency programs approved by the American Medical Association's Council on Medical Education.

J VISA: A type of visa which an Exchange Visitor may possess and which entitles a foreign medical graduate to remain in the United States for a maximum of 5 years, after which he is required to leave the country for a period of at least 2 years.

NATIONAL BOARD EXAMINATIONS: A three-part series of examinations offered to students and graduates of approved medical schools of the United States and Canada. Part I examines the candidate's knowledge of six basic medical sciences and is taken after completion of the second year of medical school. Part II examines the candidate's clinical knowledge and is taken after completion of the fourth year of medical school. Part III examines the candidate's clinical judgment and skills and is taken after successful completion of Parts I and II and a minimum of six months of internship.

P 2 HOSPITAL: Any United States hospital with approved internship and residency programs which participates in the Exchange Visitor program of the State Department.

PERMANENT RESIDENT VISA: A type of visa issued to an alien who has met the requirements for immigration which the Immigration and Naturalization Service administers. It permits the alien to remain in the United States indefinitely but does not require that he become a United States citizen, although it grants him the same responsibilities and duties which a United States citizen possesses.

FOREIGN MEDICAL GRADUATES

IN THE UNITED STATES

CHAPTER I   The Character and Role
of the Foreign Medical Graduate in the
United States Today

The records of the American Medical Association (AMA) currently contain data on 286,000 active physicians in the United States, all but 19,000 of whom are involved in direct patient care. As of January 1, 1967 there were 187,000 physicians in private practice, 45,000 serving as hospital interns, residents, or fellows, and 13,000 who were full-time members of medical faculties. The other physicians were employed in a variety of professional responsibilities, with salaried positions, including 26,000 in the Federal service.[1] Foreign medical graduates (FMGs) participated in all of these activities, and with a few exceptions were providing patient-care services.

Data from the AMA records on FMGs in medical practice are summarized in Tables B14 and B15 in the Appendix. Aside from the more than 13,000 who are in approved training programs, over 16,000 are in private medical practice; 7000 are employed by hospitals, and over 1,400 are on medical faculties; only 271 are in administrative medicine. Their income is derived from the same sources as the United States medical graduates (USMGs), although the percentage of FMGs in group practices is relatively low.[2]

Among the FMGs over 5000 are native-born United States citizens who obtained their medical degrees abroad, mostly in

Europe. They fare no better on the examination given by the Educational Council for Foreign Medical Graduates (ECFMG), (see Chapter II), which they are required to take, than do their foreign born colleagues from the same medical schools. Their professional fate is still a mystery. They have no home excepting in this country, but if they cannot pass the ECFMG examination or state licensure examinations, or both, their opportunities for medical practice in the United States are very limited. Included among the FMGs in approved training programs in 1967 were 1541 United States citizens, 506 of whom were naturalized.

Graduates of Canadian medical schools are considered the same as graduates of United States medical schools insofar as professional requirements are concerned. They are, however, subject to the same immigration regulations as are the FMGs. Canadian medical graduates are not required to take the ECFMG examination, and there are currently about 6000 of them in the United States.

The physician manpower pool in the United States has its own internal movements which are not uniform but are fairly predictable. Annual increments of physicians are derived from two basic sources: graduates of our own medical schools who become permanent members of the medical community, and graduates of foreign medical schools, who are almost equal in numbers to United States and Canadian Medical School graduates (USMGs), and who may or may not remain here permanently. We now have quite precise information about those who enter our health-care system for the first time, but comparatively vague information about those who leave it. It is estimated that every year 3800 physicians are lost through death; others retire, and an unknown number of FMGs leave the country. Several thousand USMGs enter the military service, but they return within two years with no significant domestic manpower loss during their service. A small number of physicians discontinue direct patient-care responsibilities, chiefly for

2

administration or research, and a very few abandon the profession entirely.

The uneven distribution of physicians in the country is well known. They are more heavily concentrated in certain regions and in metropolitan centers. For example, New England and the Middle Atlantic states have a ratio of physicians to population (1:550) double that of the South Central states. Furthermore, certain isolated semirural and rural areas have less than 1 physician for every 4000 people, in contrast with cities like New York that have 1 for every 400.[3] These observations become particularly meaningful in an assessment of the present and future influence of FMGs on the national health care system.

SOURCES OF INFORMATION

In this chapter we shall summarize the professional activities and characteristics of the more than 40,000 active FMGs in the United States, using the best available sources of data and pointing out, where appropriate, the need for additional data which are not collected or not reported. The most dependable source of information is found in the physician records of the AMA. Despite their remarkable usefulness, however, these records have certain limitations that must be clearly understood. The AMA depends on voluntary replies to the questionnaires it distributes and has had a very high rate of response. FMGs in approved hospital training programs, for example, are all identified. On the other hand, those in unapproved programs or in doubtful professional situations (such as patient-care responsibilities without a license to practice) may not be included in the AMA records and thus may remain a partial mystery.

The Immigration and Naturalization Service (INS) compiles complete data on physicians and other health personnel who enter the country with every kind of educational or occupational visa. The INS does not keep corresponding records on FMGs

3

who either temporarily or permanently leave the country. The INS has published figures on the number of waivers granted physicians who have J visas (Exchange Visitor), but not on those who subsequently reenter as immigrants after the mandatory two years outside the United States. An additional important deficiency is the absence of reliable information regarding the visa or citizenship status of all FMGs now in the United States. There is a similar lack of knowledge regarding the current professional activities of the several thousand native born United States citizens who obtained their medical education abroad.[4]

For many years physicians have come to the United States from other countries to pursue a full range of graduate education programs. These have included academic degree and research studies in universities, public health training, and specialized short-term courses, as well as clinical hospital training. Some FMGs have been sponsored by private foundations and others by government or international agencies, particularly the World Health Organization (WHO). The overwhelming majority, however, now emigrate to enter internships or residencies, deriving their support entirely from their own resources and from the hospitals in which they are employed. Our review of trainees will be confined to this latter group of self-sponsored FMGs now serving in United States hospitals.

CHARACTERISTICS OF FOREIGN MEDICAL GRADUATES

In this monograph we shall assiduously avoid the use of anecdotal or other material that is based solely upon impressions. Well-documented facts are especially important in any review of a controversial subject. Statistics alone, however, are highly impersonal, and their exclusive use tends to obscure the fact that the migration, education, and professional activities affect and are affected by human behavior. Physician migration is an expression of individual interests and habits which require close attention.

4

The following description is a mixture of data and personal observations that have been combined to form the profiles of some of the various types of FMGs who are currently migrating to the United States. The obvious oversimplification involved in these sketches is a sharp departure from the uses of statistical material on which this chapter otherwise depends. The chief merit of the profiles lies in their personalization of the FMGs, who otherwise are lost in tabular summaries.

The FMG now found in the majority of hospitals in this country is likely to be a little older than his USMG intern or resident colleague, is unmarried, male, and from either Asia or Latin America. He was recently graduated from a government-supported and -operated medical school which has a five-year course of studies, a skimpy budget, and a part-time faculty. He comes from a lower middle-class family which has no savings and relatively little education. He learned English as a second language, taught him by instructors for whom it was also a second language. In the United States, when he is with his compatriots or at home, he speaks his mother tongue.

His education was highly authoritarian and was occasionally interrupted by student strikes. Like many of his classmates he took an extra year to complete the requirements for his medical degree. He has taken many examinations, but the ECFMG was the first one that was both objective and comprehensive; he passed it with a minimum passing grade on the second try.

For several years he wanted to go to the United States. He has no desire to be a small-town or village doctor in his own country, but would be happy to have a clinical teaching post and a private practice in one of the major cities. To obtain that goal he is sure he must have specialty training abroad. He has not yet thought much about staying permanently in the United States, partly because he has close ties with his large family.

He learned from his older friends about hospitals in the United States that accept foreign physicians and applied to them as well as to many others. He signed an agreement with one which had on its house staff some physicians from his own country. While waiting for an appointment he had applied for a visa which was approved after several months' waiting and one change in consular officers. During his period of waiting he had a dull government dispensary job which paid a barely adequate salary.

His knowledge of hospitals in this country was limited either to the *Fact Book* on United States hospitals which the ECFMG publishes or to second-hand, fragmentary comments, and his main impressions of the United States came from movies, a few popular novels, and American tourists. He was aware of some distinction between an intern and a resident, chiefly because of the salary differential, so he was pleased to be appointed as a resident. The hospital sent no description of his future duties and he was unaware of the AMA's accreditation requirements for either the hospital or the house officer.

The hospital was located in a large Eastern city and had no full-time clinical staff. He was one of 22 interns and residents, 3 of whom were graduates of United States medical schools. When he examined a patient on his second day there it was the first time he had used English to take a medical history. Within a few days of his arrival he was given patient-care responsibilities he had never before assumed. His position at the hospital made him extremely anxious until he discovered that only rarely did anyone seem to read his histories or physical-examination notes. He quickly learned a core of routine procedures that each of the busy staff physicians wanted performed and became familiar with a number of drugs with standard dosages for common ailments. He relaxed even further when he discovered that his work would not be graded or evaluated in any specific way and that his colleagues were no better off than he was. The attending staff physicians were generally quite friendly but were too busy to supervise his work or to discuss cases with him, although some took extra time with him when they could.

The FMG is likely to remain in the United States for five years, spend time in a total of three hospitals, fail a state board examination at least once, obtain no specialty certification, and depart unhappily with the intention of returning. At home he will find many others who had a similar experience, none with a teaching position or a satisfactory income, most in government service, now regretting their loss of seniority.

This first prototypic description of the FMG may seem unwarrantedly severe. However, there are, in fact, many other individuals who came here without having passed the ECFMG, who spend little or no time in an approved hospital, who advanced from "moonlighting" to full-time practice without a license, who married to establish a "hardship" case for a permanent-resident visa, who never went home again, and who never established a sound professional base in this country.

On the other hand, there are happier examples. Our prototypic young man may have started his hospital career in an institution that has more USMGs than FMGs; he may have received an initial appointment as an intern and a later appointment as a resident in an affiliated hospital program. He may have been unusually bright, facile in languages, and he may have had a high aptitude for his specialty. Under these circumstances he still would be unlikely to achieve specialty certification or a satisfactory position at home. Rather, he might be successful in his efforts to remain in the United States, even without full hospital privileges, secure in the knowledge that he could make a comfortable living.

There are further exceptions to the foregoing examples. These include highly competent British physicians who are dissatisfied with their National Health Service, established researchers who are attracted to our splendid medical centers, and physicians from Asian British Commonwealth countries who become Members of the Royal College of Physicians before they come here, to name a few. This group is small in number, high in quality,

7

the most useful for the United States, and the most sorely missed in their own countries.

Another highly distinctive group of FMGs is made up of those who are native-born citizens of the United States. These are mostly individuals who have finished two or more years of college education in this country and have not been able to gain admission to medical school. Characteristically, they are from a large Eastern city, have academic records that were not strong enough for them to compete with other applicants to the United States medical schools where they applied, and have done correspondingly less well on the Medical College Aptitude Tests than have those whose applications were accepted. They have also applied to several medical schools in Europe, including those which usually do not accept students from countries that have their own medical schools. The institution they attend may teach in a language with which they are initially unfamiliar, although a few may have learned it from their parents or grand-parents.

These young men have very little to guide them during their studies abroad. They intend to return to the United States after graduation but have no assurance that their education will be accepted. Despite prior knowledge of the requirements, they are somewhat outraged when they find they must follow the same route for a United States hospital appointment as alien physicians from the same or other foreign schools. Most of them fail the ECFMG the first time and find their failure especially humiliating. This is only the beginning of a series of professional embarrassments which arise from the fact that their education was foreign although they are not. They have great difficulty obtaining professional acceptance from their peers and are particularly handicapped if they have continuing trouble with the ECFMG examination, not an uncommon fate for the graduates of certain medical schools. Their numbers are not large, between 300 and 400 per year, a population that is equivalent to the

8

graduating classes of three or four additional United States medical schools. In 1966–67, 1541 of the FMGs in approved hospital training programs were United States citizens. Of these, 506 were naturalized citizens and the other 1035 were native born. The Institute for International Education reported in its publication *Open Doors* (1967, page 10) that there were 2557 United States citizens studying in foreign medical schools during the past academic year. They know, and admissions committees know, that many of them would have done well in a United States medical school. Regrettably, that knowledge does nothing to alter their lives.

FOREIGN MEDICAL GRADUATE HOSPITAL TRAINEES

Of all of the available internships in the United States in 1965–66, 19 percent were filled by FMGs, 56 percent by USMGs, and the remaining 25 percent were left vacant. Of all of the available residencies, 23 percent were filled by FMGs, 59 percent by USMGs, and 18 percent remained vacant. FMGs occupied 25 percent of the internships and 32 percent of the residencies which were filled. The ratio of USMG to FMG interns was 7.4:1 in medical school-affiliated and 1.5:1 in non-affiliated hospitals.[5] These data represent a high point in the hospital employment of FMGs, a culmination of the steady increase which has occurred over the past several years. Table 1, and Table B6 in the appendix, summarize the growth over the past 15 years.

Twenty years ago the majority of physicians coming here from abroad were from European countries. Today approximately 75 percent come from the less developed nations of Africa, Asia, and Latin America. Two-thirds of the FMGs entering the United States have Exchange Visitor (J) visas which allow them a stay of five years; the other one-third have Permanent Resident (immigrant) visas.[6] They are attracted to large metropolitan centers just as are the USMGs, but they are

9

Table 1. Number of FMGs in approved internships and residencies, selected years, 1950-1967

Year	Internships filled			Residencies filled			Total FMGs	
		FMGs			FMGs			
	Total	No.	%	Total	No.	%	No.	%
1950-51	7,030	722	10	14,495	1,350	15	2,072	10
1955-56	9,603	1,859	19	21,425	4,174	21	6,033	19
1960-61	9,115	1,753	19	28,447	8,182	28	9,935	26
1965-66	9,670	2,361	24	31,898	9,133	32	11,494	28
1966-67	10,366	2,793	27	32,050	9,502	30	12,295[a]	29

Source: *JAMA, 202* (1967), 775. Used by permission of the *Journal of the American Medical Association.*

[a]There were also 2,566 FMGs who were "other trainees" in 1966-67, making the total number of FMG trainees in approved institutions 14,861.

even more concentrated than are their colleagues along the Atlantic seaboard and in few major cities like Detroit, Cleveland, and Chicago. In New Jersey, where hospitals attract an unusually low number of medical school graduates through the National Intern Matching Plan, FMGs fill 75 percent of the internships and 68 percent of the residencies, the highest percentage in the country. In some other states the total of FMGs in hospital programs is 5 percent or less.

All FMGs in approved hospitals have passed the ECFMG examination and have demonstrated some proficiency in the English language (see Chapter II). Despite the latter requirement there is a great range in language skills among, for example, native-born United States citizens or graduates of British schools and graduates of Philippine or Latin American medical schools.

First choice of hospital positions is given to USMGs rather than to FMGs. The National Intern Matching Plan fills the most attractive hospital programs with the most desirable young United States graduates. Only a few FMGs receive appointments through the Matching Plan, 406 in 1965 and 428 in 1967. With a few exceptions, FMGs are given appointments to hospitals which have been unable to attract a sufficient number of USMGs. This policy explains the observation that many hospitals are entirely dependent on FMGs and also explains the differing ratios of USMGs to FMGs in affiliated and nonaffiliated hospitals which was noted above.

Although all interns and residents, regardless of their prior education, tend to prefer similar kinds of specialty training, there are certain significant differences between FMGs and USMGs. For example, FMGs fill 46 percent of anesthesiology and 40 percent of pathology residencies, both specialties that require minimal language skill, and 27 percent of psychiatric residencies, which require maximum language skills but attract fewer USMGs. FMGs dominate general practice residencies

11

(66 percent), which appeal to very few USMGs. Only 22 percent of the USMGs who began general practice residencies in 1966–67 remained there at the end of the year.

Current patterns of residency appointments of FMGs appear to be unrelated to their medical education on their presumed responsibilities when they return home. The number appointed directly to a residency without a prior United States internship has risen rapidly in the last few years, going from 20 percent in 1964 to 30 percent in 1965 and 48 percent in 1966. In affiliated hospitals FMGs fill 67 percent of the residencies in colon and rectal surgery and 58 percent of the residencies in pediatric cardiology; in nonaffiliated hospitals they fill 45 percent of the residencies in thoracic surgery, all examples of disciplines too highly sophisticated for less developed countries.[7]

Certainly a part of the attraction which brings FMGs to the United States is the economic benefit of a comfortable, salaried position. Table B7 in the Appendix gives the range of salaries now being offered interns and residents by hospitals in this country. The average intern's salary in 1966 was $4,322, an increase of $531.58 (14 percent) over the previous year. In addition to an income that is very generous by the standards of their own countries, FMG interns and residents are provided with housing for themselves and their families and with other benefits which vary from one institution to another. In recent years there has been competition between hospitals that has led to further salary increases, particularly in those institutions that are unsuccessful in attracting USMG house officers through the reputation of their teaching programs. Some hospitals carry out aggressive programs to recruit FMGs, providing them with advances to pay for their transportation to this country and very relaxed plans for repayment. In addition there are travel bureaus that regularly inform hospitals of their services, offering to arrange the delivery of FMGs to United States hospitals. According to one account, "business is booming." [8]

Hospitals make no substantial alterations for foreign physicians in their USMG-oriented programs, except for the small number of FMGs who are brought to the United States through sponsored programs. Even those FMGs who enter directly into residencies are given patient-care responsibilities appropriate to the position they fill rather than to their scientific, clinical, or linguistic backgrounds.

The experience of FMGs varies with the hospitals in which they serve. FMGs may receive excellent training and good supervision if they are fortunate enough to obtain a position in a good teaching hospital that has only a small percentage of FMGs. If they are employed by a hospital that is primarily interested in maintaining its accreditation and in providing routine patient care through the use of house staff rather than through a program of graduate education, the FMGs may have little supervision, heavy responsibilities, and indifferent training. Indirect evidence suggests that the less favorable circumstances are not uncommon, but there have been no objective studies of the quality of graduate education FMGs receive or of the relation between their hospital experiences and their subsequent professional activities.

VISAS AND DURATION OF STAY

The duration of stay of FMG trainees in the United States has not been determined. State Department officials have the impression that those with J visas tend to remain for their full five years. The length of stay of those with immigrant visas is highly unpredictable because they can come and go easily — and not all intend to use their citizenship option. FMG trainees transfer more than do USMGs from one institution to another, as they seek situations which they consider more satisfactory either professionally or financially. At various times during their stay in this country they may marry, take state board examinations, request waivers to acquire immigrant visas without delay, and in other ways establish local ties. They may also make plans to return to their own countries (or to go to a third country like Canada), often finding formidable obstacles to repatriation in a satisfactory home assignment, that is, one appropriate to their newly acquired skills.

FOREIGN MEDICAL GRADUATE NON TRAINEES

The AMA records can account for 27,000 of the FMGs who are not now in approved hospital training programs. As indicated earlier, there are other professionally active FMGs, probably several thousand, who do not receive or do not respond to the AMA personnel questionnaire. No information is available regarding the characteristics of those who fall outside the AMA surveys; as a consequence, the data that are available are not necessarily applicable to all FMGs who are not in a training status, and very limited use can be made of the material that is available. There is a need for further studies of the professional characteristics of the entire group of FMGs, particularly those who are providing patient care either through hospital employment or in private practice.

NATIONAL DISTRIBUTION

Table 2 summarizes the location of the majority of FMGs in the United States, concentrated in ten states. The table includes data on both trainees and nontrainees and supports the impression that FMGs tend to remain in the metropolitan areas where they have received their hospital training. It can be observed from Table 2, for example, that in New York 30 percent of the total number of active physicians are FMGs. The impact of this large group on the delivery of health care is probably even greater than their numbers suggest. In all metropolitan areas there is a higher proportion of physicians in nonpatient-care activities than in the rest of the country. Of the 26,568 physicians in New York City, 1945 are not in patient-care activities.

14

Table 2. Percent of all active physicians and numbers of FMGs
in 10 states in 1966

State	Total FMGs	Percent of active physicians in state
California	2,066	6
Illinois	3,534	23
Maryland	1,518	20
Massachusetts	1,535	14
Michigan	1,696	16
New Jersey	2,360	25
New York	12,041	30
Ohio	2,681	19
Pennsylvania	1,922	11
Texas	1,041	8
Total	30,394[a]	

Source: AMA physician records.

[a]Total active FMGs in United States: 40,027; total active USMGs:
280,315

In other cities, including Philadelphia, Washington, and Baltimore, the latter group, nearly all USMGs, is even larger, com-
posing up to 15 percent of the number of total active physicians.[9] The numbers of USMGs in non-patient care activities
provide a correspondingly greater opportunity for FMGs to
provide direct patient-care services, supplementing the attractions of vacant hospital positions through which they can become qualified to practice.

Recent trends suggest some tentative changes in the national
distribution of practicing FMGs. As Table 3 indicates, data on
newly licensed physicians, specifically those representing additions to the medical profession, reveal a high percentage in

15

Table 3. Licentiates representing additions to the medical profession (1966)

State	Examinations		Reciprocity and endorsement		Total		Total licentiates
	FMGs	USMGs	FMGs	USMGs	FMGs	USMGs	
Alabama	0	61	0	5	0	66	66
Alaska	0	4	0	2	0	6	6
Arizona	1	6	0	–	1	6	7
Arkansas	0	80	0	–	0	80	80
California	46	271	0	538	46	809	855
Colorado	3	64	0	23	3	87	90
Connecticut	34	5	0	94	34	99	133
Delaware	3	9	1	0	4	9	13
District of Columbia	30	2	2	57	32	59	91
Florida	15	95	0	–	15	95	110
Georgia	13	263	0	2	13	265	278
Guam	0	–	8	–	8	0	8
Hawaii	7	7	0	16	7	23	30
Idaho	0	1	0	7	0	8	8
Illinois	77	16	0	244	77	260	337
Indiana	68	179	0	–	68	179	247
Iowa	5	99	5	3	10	102	112
Kansas	5	98	0	4	5	102	107
Kentucky	28	122	0	11	28	133	161
Louisiana	1	245	0	–	1	245	246

16

Table 3 - continued

State	Examinations		Reciprocity and endorsement		Total		Total licentiates
	FMGs	USMGs	FMGs	USMGs	FMGs	USMGs	
Maine	43	3	2	3	45	6	51
Maryland	130	148	0	90	130	238	368
Massachusetts	25	4	0	217	25	221	246
Michigan	49	283	0	1	49	284	333
Minnesota	19	141	0	112	19	253	272
Mississippi	3	100	0	5	3	105	108
Missouri	12	236	0	20	12	256	268
Montana	0	–	0	–	0	–	–
Nebraska	0	115	0	7	0	122	122
Nevada	0	–	0	–	0	–	–
New Hampshire	9	0	11	10	20	10	30
New Jersey	57	7	0	72	57	79	136
New Mexico	5	2	0	1	5	3	8
New York	197	13	17	818	214	831	1045
North Carolina	0	188	1	0	1	188	189
North Dakota	7	3	0	3	7	6	13
Ohio	16	292	1	116	17	408	425
Oklahoma	2	94	0	12	2	106	108
Oregon	4	17	0	11	4	28	32
Pennsylvania	144	66	0	353	144	419	563

Table 3 - continued

State	Examination		Reciprocity and endorsement		Total		Total licentiates
	FMGs	USMGs	FMGs	USMGs	FMGs	USMGs	
Puerto Rico	5	0	0	–	5	0	5
Rhode Island	9	1	0	6	9	7	16
South Carolina	0	69	0	4	0	73	73
South Dakota	6	10	0	1	6	11	17
Tennessee	0	134	0	7	0	141	141
Texas	100	263	1	5	101	268	369
Utah	0	26	0	16	0	42	42
Vermont	35	19	8	27	43	46	89
Virgin Islands	4	0	0	–	4	0	4
Virginia	73	147	0	30	73	177	250
Washington	34	12	0	77	34	89	123
West Virginia	5	24	0	2	5	26	31
Wisconsin	23	40	0	69	23	109	132
Wyoming	0	1	1	0	1	1	2
Total	1352	4085	58	3101	1410	7186	8596

Source: *JAMA, 200* (1967), 1061, 1071. Used by permission of the *Journal of the American Medical Association.*

certain states. In Maine, for instance, 45 out of a total of 51 licentiates representing new additions to the medical profession in 1966 were FMGs. Although this was the highest percentage of FMGs in the country, 7 out of 13 in North Dakota, 9 out of 16 in Rhode Island, 43 out of 89 in Vermont, and 20 out of 30 in New Hampshire were FMGs. The attractions of these states for FMGs may be related to the apparent shortage of health manpower. In Maine there are 905 active physicians for a population of 1 million; half of the state's physicians were graduated from medical school prior to 1945 (the national average is 39 percent), suggesting that the additional FMGs migrating into the state ultimately will have a disproportionately large responsibility for patient care. Although these trends have not yet significantly altered the distribution of FMGs, there is already evidence that they are reacting to an increased awareness of the needs for physicians in specific regions of the country.

STATE LICENSE EXAMINATIONS

What FMGs do after their training still appears to be primarily influenced by their location at the time, visa status, and specialty, and by state licensing regulations. Those with Permanent Resident visas are free to remain here indefinitely; those with J visas are supposed to leave the United States, presumably for their homelands, when their training has been completed. Both groups may write state board examinations in most states; in the last few years, thousands have done so. Those who fail an examination may continue as house officers or may be employed, as they frequently are, in other institutions, including psychiatric hospitals, that waive licensure requirements. They may also continue to take the state board examination in the same or different states.

Among the 286,000 active physicians in the AMA records, 47,500 (16.5 percent) are not licensed to practice. Of these, 18,600 (39 percent) are FMGs, almost half of the total number.

FOREIGN MEDICAL GRADUATES

Licensure data (Table 4) for some of the FMGs show striking disparities which are related to the country of education.

FMGs with permanent-resident visas who are licensed to practice have the same legal privileges and responsibilities as their colleagues trained in the United States. There are no dependable data regarding their appointments to hospital staffs, but there is evidence that in large cities many have no hospital privileges whatsoever.

EXCHANGE VISITOR VISAS

FMGs with J visas may request a waiver of the requirement that they go home for at least two years. While awaiting a decision they can remain here, thus extending their stay for several months. There has been a rapid rise in the percentage of physicians who are granted waivers, chiefly on a "hardship" basis (Appendix Table B5). Although they are required to register with the INS each January, it is extremely difficult to locate those who do not. The penalty for nonregistration is severe but is rarely imposed.[10] Those who run the mild risk of non-registration probably also avoid other kinds of registration, including the AMA's, making their identification difficult. We cannot attempt even an educated guess as to their numbers.

The object of the two-year break between Exchange-Visitor status and the acquisition of a Permanent Resident visa is to encourage repatriation and discourage the exploitation of graduate education for a change of citizenship. Government officials hope that health professionals, as well as others, will actually return to their own countries but they can only insist that they leave the United States. Many who are unable to obtain waivers go no farther than Canada, where they can readily find employment while they wait out the time for legal re-entry to this country. They have become a peculiar kind of expatriate group in limbo who describe their temporary residence as a "parking lot" status. In cities like Windsor, just across the border from

20

Table 4. Licensure status in the United States of FMGs from
certain countries

Country	Licensed	Not licensed	Percent licensed	Total
Canada[a]	4460	1262	78	5722
Argentina	297	612	33	909
Dominican Republic	162	166	49	328
Haiti	70	104	40	174
Colombia	150	446	26	596
England	741	321	70	1062
Italy	2384	427	85	2811
Switzerland	150	446	25	596
West Germany	3442	708	83	4150
Iran	229	771	23	1000
Israel	35	93	27	128
Turkey	301	290	51	591
Pakistan	13	345	4	358
India	111	1722	6	1833
Korea	119	941	11	1060
Philippines	761	4295	15	5056
Taiwan	33	407	8	440
Thailand	16	586	3	602

Source: AMA physician records.

[a]Graduates of Canadian medical schools are considered the same as USMGs
by the AMA's Council on Medical Education. They are considered as FMGs
by the INS.

Detroit, they form a unique colony which is composed chiefly of physicians and nurses that has its own assets, not the least of which is an encyclopedic knowledge of immigration and employment procedures.

PERSISTING PHYSICIAN SHORTAGES

There is abundant evidence that shortages of physicians in the United States will persist, as will shortages of nurses and other members of the health professions. Estimates vary on the exact numbers needed to meet national health care demands but there is agreement on a clearly predictable shortage beyond the next decade. In June 1967, the AMA concluded that there is a "critical need for more physicians, for a better distribution of physician resources, and for allied health personnel in all categories . . . In spite of the fact that medical school output has been increasing steadily, and that such a trend will no doubt continue during the ensuing years, the resulting increment will probably not suffice to resolve the physician manpower problems. While increasing utilization of allied health personnel in roles supportive to the physician and modifications in the organization and delivery of health services may influence future requirements for physician manpower, there is little evidence that these measures will satisfy the foreseeable rising demand for physicians or rectify existent and anticipated shortages in this field." [11]

Raw numerical estimates are not very satisfactory statistical tools for measuring health manpower needs, but they have some use as general indicators. The Department of Labor, using standard employment criteria, has reported a current shortage of 100,000 physicians in the United States.[12] The Public Health Service's data indicate a need for 400,000 physicians by 1975, approximately 110,000 more than we now have.[13] The National Advisory Commission on Health Manpower, in its November 1967 report to President Johnson, said: "There is currently a shortage of physicians and this shortage will worsen in relation to growing demand." The Commission, however, went on to say: "While the need to increase the production of physicians above presently planned levels is clear, the extent of the increase required is uncertain." [14]

Darley and Somers [15] re-examined the goal established by the 1959 Surgeon General's Consultant Group on Medical Education in the light of subsequent and planned increases in medical school output. They concluded that by 1975 we will fall 50 percent short of the desired level of physician production, thus accentuating the already existing shortages.

A critical analysis of health manpower needs has been done by Rashi Fein [16] through the use of more functional economic tools. He has measured physicians' services, rather than the number of physicians, against the existing and projected demands for those services. He took into account such factors as demographic and socioeconomic changes, alterations in the organization of medical care, the introduction of new types of personnel, and changing methods of payment for health care services. He predicted a total increase in demand for health services by 1975 of 22–26 percent (but indicated that it might rise by 1980 to as much as 35–40 percent). The increase in physicians' services by 1975, according to his calculations, will be only 19 percent with continued importations of FMGs and 13 percent without them. Even with a marked rise in productivity by the health professions there would remain a gap which could not be filled by the planned output of medical schools. It should be noted that his method of analysis had to assume that the present balance between supply and demand for health services is a desirable level to maintain. As noted above, however, this appears not to be the case.

The physician shortage has already produced some response on the part of the medical school in this country. Graduates of medical schools in the United States increased from 7000 in

23

1955 to 7600 in 1965. Through expansion of existing institutions and an unprecedented increase in the number of new schools, their total output is expected to reach 10,000 by 1975. Despite this rapid growth, the overall effect of the additional graduates on a national physician pool of 286,000 will be insufficient to meet more rapidly growing demands. If the present supply of FMGs to the United States were suddenly cut off, the total number of new graduates entering the health care system in 1965 would be 25–30 percent less than it is now.

Hospitals have long been aware of these shortages. For several years the supply of USMGs has been much less than the number required to fill all of the approved internships and residencies. In 1965–66 there were 13,600 available internships and only 7573 USMGs, leaving 6000 vacancies, 44 percent of which were filled by FMGs. USMGs were available to fill 22,500 of the 39,000 residencies offered; 56 percent of the remaining 16,500 were filled by FMGs, leaving 6027 vacant.[17] With the planned expansion of medical facilities, including those associated with the new medical schools, the opportunities for both internships and residencies will increase proportionately. Under the most optimistic conditions, there will not be enough USMGs by 1975 to meet the hospital staff needs of 1965, much less those that will have been added in the intervening decade. From the viewpoint of the employment market, the United States thus will long remain attractive for foreign medical graduates.

CHAPTER II   The Educational Council for

Foreign Medical Graduates

The Educational Council for Foreign Medical Graduates (ECFMG) is a non-governmental regulatory body, created and supported by voluntary medical organizations in the United States. It has no counterpart elsewhere in the world. The responsibilities and functions of the ECFMG are an extension of the whole system of control that physicians and hospitals have chosen to impose upon themselves; the vital role it plays in physician migration will become apparent in this chapter. To assure a fuller understanding of this unique institution, more detailed information is included in Appendix A.

The formation of the ECFMG was a logical outgrowth of the other regulatory procedures which lead to hospital approval and accreditation. The AMA, through its Council on Education, determines the acceptability of programs which provide graduate medical education; it also determines the qualifications required of the physicians admitted as interns and residents to those programs. State boards of medical examiners in turn utilize the AMA's published lists of approved institutions for their own legal requirements, thereby converting privately sponsored regulations into official regulations. Through this chain of events, and others which are similar, the AMA has changed from a purely professional body into a quasi-public agency, serving both its functions satisfactorily.

FMGs have raised additional problems, including the need

for measurements of FMGs' fitness for graduate education in the United States. By choosing an evaluation process based on tests which have been taken by USMGs to measure the FMGs' medical knowledge, the AMA and other voluntary medical organizations have assured hospitals and the patients they serve that FMGs have a level of professional skills which we require of our own graduates. More explicitly, those FMGs who are certified by the ECFMG are thereby made fully acceptable for graduate medical education in any approved program in the United States. The review of the ECFMG and its activities that follows will consider the implications of its program for medical education and the delivery of health care in the United States.

MEDICAL SCHOOLS AND ACCREDITING PROCEDURES

The 286,000 active physicians in the United States today represent scores of specialties and subspecialties and are graduates of hundreds of medical schools. Most have had a sound education; some have not. Those who are graduates of United States medical schools began their careers with known professional qualities because this country maintains a carefully designed, though voluntary, system of medical school review and accreditation which has worked quite well. Special studies are constantly conducted in an effort to improve the quality of medical education, and evaluative procedures are regularly reviewed to assure the highest possible standards in this country's institutions.

Graduation from a United States medical school is considered prima facie evidence of professional competence for admission to programs for postgraduate training, for medical military service, for eligibility for licensure in any of our states, and in general for acceptance as a member of the medical community. This situation is possible because of the high minimum standards for medical education maintained through the joint efforts of the American Medical Association and the Association of

American Medical Colleges (AAMC), which are given the responsibility through their Liaison Committee for the whole process of medical school accreditation. So successful has been their procedure of regular visits and reviews that their recommendations have been fully accepted by the medical profession, the academic world, and both state and federal agencies. Thus, all of the United States medical schools, despite marked differences in curricula, size, admission policies, and overall orientation, have a common point of reference: the essential quality and characteristics of their graduates are known.

No similar procedures are conducted on a worldwide basis. The World Health Organization (WHO) assembles raw data and periodically publishes a *World Directory of Medical Schools*, which describes the salient features of undergraduate medical education in the countries that have medical schools. WHO makes no attempt, however, to classify or accredit these schools, and no firm international criteria of acceptable medical standards have ever been established.

From 1950 to 1960 the Council on Medical Education and Hospitals of the AMA and the Executive Council of the AAMC published lists of foreign medical schools that they felt were equivalent in quality to those in the United States. The lists were intended as guides in the selection of FMGs for service in United States hospitals, but it soon became apparent that neither organization had adequate evaluative procedures for medical schools in other countries and the publication was abandoned.

MEDICAL GRADUATES IN THE UNITED STATES

Given the lack of evaluation procedure for foreign medical schools, there are now two types of medical school graduates in the United States: one of known and the other of uncertain quality. The USMG has been educated in a system that our medical profession fully understands and over which it exercises adequate control. The FMG obtained his medical degree in a system with which the United States has little or no familiarity and over which it can exercise absolutely no control. The number of FMGs who have entered the United States health care system annually during the past five years has almost equaled the annual number of graduates from United States medical schools. This balance between USMGs and FMGs is, however, affected by the unknown number of FMGs who annually depart from the United States.

REGULATORY MECHANISMS

There are two regulatory mechanisms that control the admission of physicians into the health manpower system in the United States. One is the result of the evolutionary process of United States medical education, and governs the standards for graduation from a United States medical school, the requirements for internships and residencies, and the stipulations for medical licensure. The other allows FMGs to enter the United States medical profession on the basis of passing a qualifying examination, the presentation of bona fide credentials, and the payment of a fee. The former is the entire United States medical education system; the latter is the ECFMG.

Any physician whose medical degree has been conferred by a school of medicine outside of the United States, Canada, or Puerto Rico is considered a "foreign medical graduate." This definition applies equally to United States citizens who receive their medical education abroad and to citizens of other countries who have been educated in any of the more than 700 medical schools of the world. It is estimated that approximately 350 United States citizens annually apply to write the ECFMG examination.[1]

If a graduate of a foreign medical school wishes to come to the United States for approved postgraduate training, it is necessary for him to have certification from the ECFMG. The American Hospital Association (AHA) requires that all FMGs

28

in accredited and registered hospitals have either full and unrestricted licenses to practice in this country or ECFMG certification. Since 1960 the AMA has required ECFMG certification for FMGs who receive appointment into approved internship or residency programs, unless the FMGs have full and unrestricted license to practice medicine in the states or territories. While every state and territory belonging to the United States has the right to establish its own conditions for medical practice within its borders, almost all have accepted the necessity of ECFMG certification before an FMG is admitted for licensure or for graduate training in an approved hospital.

Forty-three of the 55 states and territorial jurisdictions in the United States require that physicians trained in foreign countries other than Canada pass the ECFMG examination as a prerequisite to admission to their licensing examinations. Of the twelve remaining jurisdictions, Arkansas, Louisiana, and Nevada accept no FMGs. The remaining nine states and territories impose a range of other restrictions. For example, California requires a two-year internship in an approved United States hospital. Delaware requires a one-year residency period in that state. Illinois will issue a limited license, pursuant to regulations established by the Illinois State Board of Examiners. Indiana requires two years of postgraduate training in an approved United States hospital and United States citizenship. Kansas has stipulations governing the type of evidence an FMG must present, such as his college curriculum, diploma, and license. Massachusetts law states that an FMG must furnish documentary evidence that his education is equivalent to that of graduates of medical schools in this country and also that he passed the National Board Examination. In New Jersey an FMG must present evidence of having had at least three years of training in a hospital approved by the State Board. In New York the Board of Regents maintains a list of accepted foreign medical schools, and graduates of schools not on this list may be required to take additional training in an approved United States hospital. Also, the ECFMG Examination "or its equivalent" is required. Puerto Rico requires full citizenship, and the Virgin Islands require a six-month residency period.[2]

As a result of these regulations, any FMG who wishes to receive training in an approved hospital or be admitted for a licensure examination in the United States or its territories must, either directly or indirectly, have ECFMG certification. (The conflict between these requirements and the December 1965 Department of Labor ruling on the issuance of visas is discussed in Chapter IV.)

Certification by the ECFMG is a rather complicated procedure for an FMG. Before receiving a Standard Certificate an FMG must go through several processes. He must present his credentials for validation and must show that he has completed a minimum of four accredited years in a medical school that is listed in the *World Directory of Medical Schools*, that he successfully completed the full medical curriculum of the school he attended, and that he received an accepted degree from that school. In many countries he must also be fully qualified to practice medicine.

After an FMG's medical credentials have been established, he must then pass an examination which the ECFMG administers twice yearly in centers throughout the United States and abroad. The examination lasts one day and consists of two parts, one that examines the FMG's medical knowledge with 360 multiple-choice questions and one that is designed to test his knowledge of English.

A score of 75 percent must be obtained by the FMG to receive a passing grade on the medical portion of the ECFMG examination. A successful candidate must also pass the English portion of the ECFMG examination. Armed with a passing score of 75 percent or more, successful completion of the English examination, and validation of all his medical credentials, an FMG may then apply at the nearest United States consulate in his country for a visa to come to the United States for advanced training, or for another examination if he wishes to enter medical practice. In spite of this formidable array of requirements and paper work, each year FMG's by the thousands seek ECFMG certification. They courageously wade through the tangle of regulations and patiently await the results of accreditation and visa approvals. It usually takes several months to get all of the FMGs' papers in order, and can take several years. Nonetheless, the ultimate prize of a house staff position in a United States hospital, coupled with the advantages of training in the world's best medical facilities and a nice pay check every month, compel them to make the efforts.

The first ECFMG examination, given in March 1958, was taken by 298 FMGs, of whom 151 (51 percent) passed. The following year the number taking the examination had quadrupled, and in 1960 a period of phenomenal growth began. That year a total of 14,768 wrote the examination; since 1963 an average of 18,700 FMGs have annually taken the examination. The passing rate for those taking it for the first time ranges between 30 and 45 percent. There is no limitation on the number of times an FMG may take the examination, and the number of repeaters each year exceeds the total taking it for the first time. With extraordinary tenacity of purpose, approximately 60 percent of those who take it ultimately pass the ECFMG examination and come to the United States for training. The total figures for the past nine years are shown in Tables 5 and 6.

EXPANDED PURPOSES OF THE ECFMG

Owing to the totally unexpected increase in the number of applicants for the ECFMG examination and the concomitant responsibilities which this volume of FMGs presented to the United States medical community, a Conference on International Education in Medicine was convened in Washington in Decem-

32

Table 5. Number of FMGs taking the ECFMG Examination, 1958-1966

Examination Centers	1958	1959	1960	1961	1962	1963	1964	1965	1966
Total	1,005	4,840	14,768	14,222	14,535	19,130	18,511	18,337	18,988
Domestic	868	3,629	12,217	8,530	5,913	6,054	5,712	5,078	3,925
Foreign	137	1,211	2,551	5,692	8,622	13,259	12,799	13,259	15,063

Source: ECFMG *Annual Report*, 1966, p. 9. Used by permission of the ECFMG.

Table 6. Performance of FMGs on ECFMG examinations,
1961-1966

Year	Number of candidates	Percent scoring 75 percent or higher
1961	14,222	37.8
1962	14,535	41.7
1963	19,130	31.6
1964	18,511	36.8
1965	18,337	42.1
1966	18,988	41.2

Source: ECFMG *Annual Reports,* 1961-1966. Used by permission of the
ECFMG.

ber 1960. The purpose of the conference was to discuss ways
in which the medical profession, as well as public and other
private sectors, could meet the crisis.

A special Steering Committee was appointed to advise the
ECFMG (See Appendix A) on methods for implementing its
original purposes and for expanding its activities. As a result
of the Steering Committee's proposals, in 1962 the Board of
Trustees of the ECFMG authorized a revised statement of its
purposes, and these goals were outlined for the first time in the
Annual Report for 1962 of the ECFMG.

At the same time the Board of Trustees decided that it would
reserve the right to use its own judgment with regard to the
precise scope and details of the ECFMG's program. With this
reservation, the ECFMG published the following statement of
its primary functions:

1. To promote the advanced study of medicine in the United
    States of America by graduates of foreign medical schools
    and thereby to assist those graduates in raised the level
    of medical care and medical education of other countries.

33

2. To expand, for graduates of foreign medical schools, the educational opportunity in hospitals in the United States.
3. To serve the public interest by a program of education, testing and evaluation of foreign trained physicians which will help assure the public that such physicians are properly qualified to assume responsibility for the care of patients as interns or residents in hospitals in the United States.
4. To evaluate the educational qualifications and medical training of foreign physicians who desire to further their education in the United States and with respect thereto, to verify credentials, to arrange, supervise and conduct examinations to determine the readiness of such individuals to benefit from education as interns or residents in United States hospitals.
5. To disseminate information and data among graduates of foreign medical schools relating to the programs, requirements and procedures for residents and interns in hospitals in the United States and thereby enable them to prepare to obtain maximum benefit from these hospital programs.
6. To assist in the continued improvement of the medical educational programs and standards of hospitals in the United States.[3]

Among the ECFMG's major accomplishments has been success in resolving many administrative and procedural problems with a program which has experienced unexpected growth. Following a 1962 questionnaire sent to a sample of FMG interns and residents, the ECFMG published a *Handbook for Foreign Medical Graduates* which has been in circulation since 1965. They have also maintained close liaison with many of the national and international organizations that are concerned with international medical education. The ECFMG has also developed techniques for the evaluation of credentials and the assessment of educational qualifications. During 1966, it supported studies of selected FMG interns and residents conducted by the Hospital Research and Educational Trust of New Jersey and New York University.

34

In a speech presented at the Annual Examination Institute of the Federation of State Medical Boards of the United States, Dr. Halsey Hunt, Executive Director of the ECFMG, stated that the ECFMG had faced three major problems: the mechanics of "handling an unexpectedly large program," the "difficulties of determining what are the proper and equitable educational requirements," and the task of "getting the understanding and cooperation of U.S. hospitals." [4]

The Council continues to have even larger problems that cannot be resolved merely through administrative procedures. They represent conflicts between intent and practice, involving the examination procedure, the quality of the FMG who is certified, the needs of hospitals for interns and residents, and the student-physicians who need training relevant to their backgrounds and professional ambitions.

In its 1962 statement of basic goals, the ECFMG publicly took cognizance of the fact that FMGs would provide direct patient care. Point three of its statement of purpose says that the ECFMG will seek "to serve public interest by a program of education, testing, and evaluation of foreign physicians . . . to assume responsibility for the care of patients . . . in hospitals in the U.S." In its *Annual Report* for 1965 the ECFMG said: "It must not be assumed, however, that passing the ECFMG means the same as passing the National Board examinations. Questions that have been judged to be very difficult for American graduates have not been included in the ECFMG examinations . . . National Board Certification requires a total of five days; the ECFMG is completed in one day, and on this day six and one-half hours are allowed for a number of questions that would have had an allowance of four hours for National Board candidates. The scores are designed to be equivalent with respect to those elements of medical knowledge generally accepted on a world-wide basis." [5] The difference between the USMGs and

35

FMGs in performance on their examinations is shown on Charts 1 and 2.

A recent AMA editorial noted the present disparity between the stated purpose of the ECFMG and the realities of the prevailing situation in the United States. Entitled "The Quality of Medicine is Strained," the editorial commented that the ECFMG examination "consists of questions provided by the National Board of Medical Examiners after removal of questions that have been shown to be difficult to answer in the National Board Examinations to which graduates of U.S. schools submit themselves . . . A double standard exists, for part of which the medical profession is responsible." [6] In the same issue, however, the AMA issued the following statement: "This is the current recommendation of the Council on Medical Education of the AMA and the Executive Council of the AAMC that agencies in the U.S. concerned with the medical qualifications of graduates of foreign medical schools consider certification by the ECFMG as evidence that the recipients of such certification have medical knowledge at least comparative with the minimum expected of approved schools in the United States and Canada." [7]

A fundamental issue that the ECFMG needs to resolve in its qualifying examinations is the conflict between original purpose and present practices. The examination that was designed to identify FMGs who could benefit from special graduate education programs is actually being used by hospitals and the FMGs to select substitutes for USMGs who are in short supply. It is made up of carefully selected questions that are both permissive and challenging, explicitly separating the requirements for FMGs from those for USMGs. At the point of application, in the hospitals, this differentiation is lost.

Some of the difficulties arise from the process of FMG selection, others from the kind of education the FMGs receive in this country. Simply stated, there are two kinds of FMGs; those who will return to their own countries and those who will remain

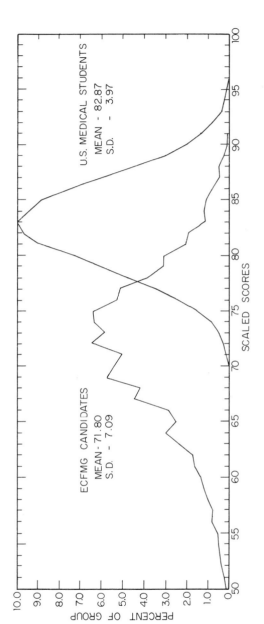

CHART 1. Percentage Distribution — ECFMG Examination, March 24, 1965. Actual Distribution of ECFMG Candidates; Expected Distribution of U.S. Medical Students

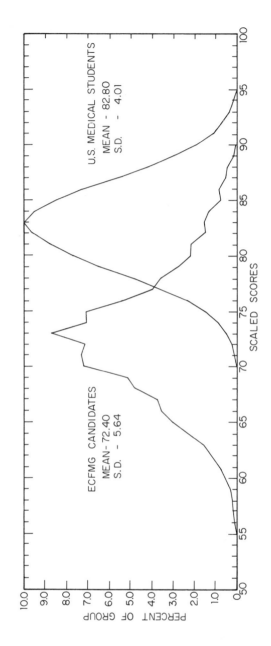

CHART 2. Percentage Distribution — ECFMG Examination, September 15, 1965. Actual Distribution of ECFMG Candidates; Expected Distribution of U.S. Medical Students

Source: ECFMG *Annual Report*, 1966, p. 12. Used by permission of the ECFMG.

permanently in the United States. The method of selection for appointment to a hospital, usually for a self-sponsored individual from a less developed country, makes no distinction whatsoever between these two future careers. The technical qualifications required of the two groups, and their educational needs, are fundamentally different.

Those who come to the United States to acquire knowledge and skills applicable in their countries of origin should be chosen and educated in accordance with their future activities. For these individuals the standards of practice and health care of their own countries should prevail. They should not be impeded by the need to participate temporarily or permanently in the delivery of health care through the highly sophisticated system that the United States enjoys.

When they return home, they should have empathy for the needs of their own people and should have gained a greater capacity to improve local health care through whatever assignments they accept. If the FMGs' United States programs are carefully planned and carried out with their specific needs and future career plans in mind, they will be able to adapt the knowledge gained here to meet the needs of their home countries.

There presently is no method for discriminating between the two groups of FMG physicians. They come on either type of visa, take the same ECFMG examinations, remain here for the same period of time, seek the same kind of certificates of competence, and participate in the same kinds of training. Because the ECFMG was planned around the needs of those who presumably will go home again, the requirements for FMGs are not the same as those for USMGs. As a consequence, the quality of health care provided during the FMGs' hospital assignments or thereafter may not be what the patient expects and deserves. Training programs that are specifically designed for the USMG and the community he serves remain unaltered for the FMG no matter where he comes from or where he is going. Within 24 hours of his arrival the FMG may be thrust into a hospital routine for which he is unprepared, and from which he will emerge months or years later altered personally and professionally in ways that have never been evaluated. A highly motivated, conscientious young physician will search in vain for training that will prepare him for the patient care needs of his own people in Asia or Latin America. Instead he will find himself increasingly tempted to forget the reasons for his emigration as the opportunities broaden for him to remain here permanently, or as his home ties begin to loosen after years of study in the United States.

The ECFMG examination adequately identifies physicians for specialized training programs in the United States that do not exist, and inadequately identifies physicians for training programs that in fact they do enter and for patient care responsibilities that they inevitably assume. In neither case is the FMG or the community well served. The country of origin is denied the physician's services either temporarily or permanently, and at best receives in return a physician whose time was partly wasted. The United States gets a physician who has been educated in a medical school which does not meet our standards, trained in hospitals here that have done little to correct his deficiencies, and who finally leaves the hospital willing but still doubtfully prepared to practice medicine somewhere in this country.

Unfortunately, the ECFMG is wrestling with problems that considerably exceed the capacities of any one organization. It is recognized as the United States medical community's official organ and a channel through which FMGs gain entrance into this country, but it has no explicit legal authority. It has been successful in making ECFMG certification a prerequisite for entrance into an approved internship or residency program, or for admission before most state licensing boards; but it has been partly circumvented by a Labor Department ruling that was based upon considerations other than United States standards for medical competence. The remainder of the United States medical community, while interested in the ways in which the ECFMG meets its responsibilities, has not yet fully defined the problem nor worked vigorously through the ECFMG toward its resolution.

The ECFMG wishes to serve the public interest but cannot control the nature of FMG activities in United States hospitals. It would be willing to serve as counselor and guide for FMGs, but has had little time or organization for these activities. It tests the FMG's ability and competence in the English language to evaluate his readiness for training in a United States hospital, but does so with a 50-item multiple choice examination. It is genuinely interested in performing an international service but is often inadvertently a national employment agency for United States hospitals.

If reasonable order is to arise out of the present confusion, the ECFMG, with the advice and assistance of the United States medical community, must begin to cope with a situation that it did not create, but which it has helped to foster. It has thus far enunciated some sound, basic goals and proceeded to deal primarily with an enormous amount of paper work. Its major weaknesses are the result of policy decisions made early in its history, before the occurrence of events that have challenged the wisdom of these decisions. No one could have predicted the unprecedented migration of FMGs that has so greatly affected systems of postgraduate medical education and health care in the United States. Whether errors have arisen from expedient or careful judgments, they can be rectified only by careful, thoughtful revisions. These revisions will be the responsibility of the Board of Trustees of the ECFMG, on whom all effective action depends. The only alternative to such action is to state boldly that the United States now accepts two levels of medical practice provided by two different types of physicians who have two distinctly different levels of competence.

The quasi-public character of the ECFMG has attracted less attention than have its purely professional activities. Some examples of the former are worth noting. The ECFMG has de facto modified the United States immigration laws by persuading the Department of State to include ECFMG certification as one of the requirements for issuance of a visa to an FMG. In turn, government officials have not insisted on reviewing the merits of the examination or the implications of this procedure although the Department of Labor has chosen to ignore the ECFMG examination. The records of the ECFMG are not all subject to public scrutiny and some of them are kept confidential, subject only to the judgment of the staff.

By setting up examination centers throughout the world, the ECFMG has provided an invaluable service to those physicians who would otherwise be unable to qualify for a hospital appointment in the United States. However, this action was not without other implications. As accessibility to the examination rose, so did the rate of migration. This has elevated to a higher level concern about brain drain as an international issue, a concern sometimes expressed by harsh accusations against the United States.

Medical leaders in other countries are aware of the unsatisfactory training which many FMGs receive in this country. The ECFMG and its Trustee members, by implication, are blamed. Physicians who spend several years in the United States in what later appears to have been a misguided venture represent a policy failure to which the ECFMG, however unwittingly, has contributed. When these are rare events they may not be troublesome; when they are common they become matters of concern. In either case, there is no requirement for accountability regarding what has clearly become a public policy issue.

This is not to suggest that the ECFMG has not worked closely with United States government and foreign officials, but the fact remains that it is not subject to any external controls or review. To the rest of the world the examination which is given through the offices of the United States Information Agency (USIA) in Embassies and Consulates, presented as a requirement for issuance of a visa, is seen as an official government action. When India disallowed the examination to be given in its cities the action was taken by the government of India following diplomatic exchanges. When the United Arab Republic recently agreed to let its physicians take the examination there for the first time it was a manifestation of improved United States-Egyptian relationships; these were abruptly altered during the UAR's conflict with Israel. Fortunately, the latter event occurred before rather than during the time the examination was to have been given.

Obviously, such issues as migration, graduate education, health manpower needs, and immigration policies are much larger than the issues affecting foreign medical graduates and the ECFMG. Furthermore, the ECFMG is not qualified to serve a diplomatic function that is reserved for the Department of State and its counterparts in other countries. There may very well be a need, therefore, to distinguish more clearly between the areas of responsibility that are germane to the competence of voluntary professional bodies in the United States and those that go beyond their reasonable purview. Even if the process of selection of FMGs is to continue as a relaxed collaboration between private and governmental agencies there should be a better measure of the full consequence of that collaboration.

Decisions affecting public policy will consistently be more prudent when they are based on a full range of human skills and a sound awareness of the circumstances bearing on those decisions. Even greater wisdom will emerge when there is continuing and recognizable responsibility for the end results. The Council and its Trustees may prefer to confine themselves to those purely professional actions for which their experiences so well qualify them. If so, they also may find it necessary to seek guidance and share responsibilities with other public and private groups before rather than after they have been forced into less familiar paths.

CHAPTER III Professional Qualities of

Foreign Medical Graduates

We have approached this section of the monograph with considerable caution. Despite the great advances made in examining techniques through the effort of such organizations as the Educational Testing Service and the National Board of Medical Examiners, measurements of professional competence in any discipline are notoriously hazardous. Theoretically, it might be best to judge competence by continuous testing and review of the results achieved in the practical application of acquired knowledge. For the individual physician such a procedure would also mean a long-term analysis of how effective he has been in keeping his patients well, in curing the ailing, or in easing the incurable. Even this impractical goal would be unsatisfactory in most cases, and impossible in many. We would prefer to judge the physician before he is completely free to practice his skill.

For generations, the United States has relied heavily on the quality of medical education provided through its accredited institutions, and it is assumed by the medical profession and the public that this country's medical school graduates meet the established criteria for professional competence. Any physician who has received his medical degree and wishes to practice in the United States must have been granted his degree by a medical school fully approved by both the AMA and the Association of American Medical Colleges (AAMC). Decades have passed since physicians could be licensed after only an apprenticeship training, and for over twenty years there have been no "Class B" medical schools. All institutions must meet the high minimum standards set by the medical profession through its voluntary system.

The quality of medical education that has been established and carefully supervised in this country has had a strong influence on the state licensure examinations. Individual states and territorial licensing bodies continue to exercise the traditional privilege of determining the suitability of any physician who wishes to practice medicine under their jurisdictions, but the examination itself may be almost a technical formality. A state resident who has obtained an M.D. degree from his state university almost invariably passes that state's licensure examination. Reciprocity between states is common, and there is nearly universal acceptance of the National Board Examination that is now preferred to the State Board Examinations by the majority of United States graduates.

A license to practice medicine grants the associated privileges and responsibilities in perpetuity. There is no reexamination and no requirement for any kind of subsequent reaccreditation. Furthermore, interns and residents are not required to pass any kind of test during their training to prove even minimal knowledge of their chosen subjects, even though their graduate education may last longer than did their undergraduate years. American Board certification in the various specialties is obtained only after the candidate passes very demanding examinations, but it is not a statutory requirement for specialty practice, and it is taken at least one or two years after the completion of the physician's graduate education program.

Foreign medical graduates who migrate to the United States have completely bypassed the most effective measurement of professional competence we know and use: graduation from a United States medical school. As a consequence, we must depend heavily in this chapter upon other available methods of evaluation, recognizing their limitations and applying only what appears to be valid.

FOREIGN MEDICAL SCHOOLS

Despite the lack of completely reliable, objective standards, there is some value to be derived from a short review of the medical schools from which most of the FMGs migrating to the United States were graduated. Although the comments that follow apply primarily to institutions in Asia, Africa, and Latin America, there are on those continents outstanding institutions which are notable exceptions to those which are described in this chapter. Certainly such centers of excellence are to be found, for example, in Japan, Israel, Lebanon, South Africa, and Turkey.

It was pointed out in Chapter II that in 1960 the AMA and the AAMC abandoned a decade of efforts to judge the medical schools of other countries. They now depend upon the ECFMG examination, which treats alike all graduates of the 700 or more medical schools located outside the United States and Canada. That the schools are not alike is obvious. Medical education in England, Sweden, Switzerland, and other Western European countries is representative of the best in the world, whereas the less developed countries in general cannot approach these high levels.

The differences begin early. Most of our FMGs come from schools that require no more than two years of premedical education, in contrast to the United States' three or four years. Furthermore, the FMGs' premedical education occurs at an age when our students are still in high school, and the FMGs' scientific studies are confined to rather simple instruction in physics, chemistry, and biology, with little or no mathematics. Despite recent efforts by the Peace Corps, the State Department, and other agencies to improve the teaching of science in less developed countries, the quality of instruction falls below what the medical students of more affluent countries now receive in secondary school. Students in the United States usually go on to obtain undergraduate degrees before entering medical school. As a consequence, they are three to four years older than their counterparts abroad and have already acquired an understanding of the fundamentals of those subjects on which the medical sciences are based.

Most foreign medical schools require five years of course work, whereas four are required in the United States; but foreign internships are not always a routine period of additional education as they are in this country. Foreign medical schools range in size from a total enrollment of 24 at the *Geneeskundige School* in Paramaribo, Surinam to 7825 at the *Institut de Medicina si Farmacie* in Bucharest, Romania.[1] Although they are usually free-standing institutions without the close university relation which we in this country greatly prefer, they are dominated by the academic practices of the local system of higher education. They use much more didactic teaching than do medical schools in the United States, and in many countries what is taught is considerably less important than what will be demanded of students by the rigid examination system.

There are marked variations in the academic practices of foreign medical schools. Some countries insist that all students who have obtained passing marks in the premedical courses required for medical school entrance should be admitted regardless of their level of scholastic achievement. The medical schools may also allow students to continue attending courses even after repeated failures, thus adding further to the sizes of overburdened classes. In general, the faculty-student ratio is much lower than in the United States or in Europe; in actuality, it is even lower than the statistics indicate because it is a custom for faculty members in less developed countries to spend most of their time in private practice. Salary levels for both clinical and basic science teachers are frequently so meager that this practice is a condition of survival.

Many foreign medical schools have very limited financial support. Laboratories are often ill-equipped and poorly maintained, libraries are so inadequate they have been of special concern to the World Health Organization, and textbooks for both students and teachers are frequently in short supply or not available at all. In Asia and Africa the language used for teaching may not be the mother tongue of either the students or the faculty; if the national language is used there are almost no current textbooks or journals excepting those written in English or, less frequently, in French. Latin American schools are somewhat better off than many others because of the greater availability of Spanish-language material. In any case, communication with patients must be in whatever vernacular the patient uses, translated into one or more tongues as the occasion demands. Research is not a significant faculty activity, because both talent and supporting funds for research are rare luxuries.

Most foreign medical schools are fully supported by their government and commonly are a part of the civil service system. In less developed countries there are severe shortages of nurses, drugs, and diagnostic equipment, and lower levels of personnel are so poorly trained and poorly paid that they cannot provide minimal helping services. Some medical schools, for example in the Philippines, are private profit-making institutions, deriving almost all of their funds from student tuitions which must not only meet institutional expenses but also show a return to the stockholders.

We must again stress the fact that there are striking exceptions to the preceding statements. On the other hand, there are few if any foreign medical schools in less developed countries that are as well endowed as the least endowed medical schools in the United States. Our schools receive greater financial support, have superior physical and scientific facilities, larger full-time faculties with smaller student bodies, and more demanding academic programs. In the United States, moreover, the medical student's hours of work are longer, vacations shorter, and clinical and laboratory experience more extensive.

Under the circumstances, it is at least prudent to inquire into the relative professional competence of the FMG and the USMG, with specific reference to the roles they play in our educational and health care systems.

THE PERFORMANCE OF FMGS AS INTERNS AND RESIDENTS

In 1967 the authors conducted a study of the professional quality of FMGs for the Association of American Medical Colleges and the National Advisory Commission on Health Manpower.[2] The survey was confined to FMGs who were serving as interns and residents in approved United States hospital training programs. The evaluation was based on a direct comparison between FMGs and USMGs who were on the same hospital service, under the same supervision, receiving the same training, and with similar patient care responsibilities. Evaluations of individual professional competence were made by those members of the teaching staff who were in charge of the internship or specialty services of the FMG and USMG. A total of 296 FMGs and 166 USMGs were evaluated in the 156 hospitals that were surveyed. The larger number of FMGs represents the participation of hospitals that had only FMGs on their house staffs. Hospitals that filled all their positions with USMGs were not included in the study. Hospitals were otherwise selected by random sampling, and the individuals studied were selected by us, rather than by the participating hospitals, on a proportionally representative basis.

Professional competence was judged by responses to fifteen questions which covered the following factors: (1) acclimatization to new environment and duties; (2) ability to accept discipline; (3) competence in general house officer's duties;

49

(4) ability to take a medical history; (5) ability to perform a physical examination; (6) knowledge of basic medical sciences; (7) quality of relations with patients; (8) character of personal relations in hospital; (9) character of professional relations with staff in hospital; (10) skill in the use of libraries; (11) need for supervision in patient care; (12) rate of learning; (13) effect on teaching functions of staff; (14) capacity for independent learning; (15) fitness for medical practice in the local community. The results of these evaluations are shown in Table 7.

With the exception of the questions relating to personal characteristics, such as acclimatization and acceptance of discipline, the 271 evaluators rated the FMGs significantly lower in competence than their USMG counterparts. This statistically significant difference emerged on every question that measured professional skills and verified the judgment that, as a group, the FMGs have a limited capacity for independent learning, require (but do not receive) close supervision, and are predictably less suitable than are the USMGs to become members of the local medical community. FMGs achieved the same rating whether or not they were employed by hospitals that also had USMG interns and residents.

Individual exceptions appeared but were rather rare. The portion of the study in which 156 hospital administrators responded to more general questions revealed a general administrative awareness of wide differences among FMGs, who usually also have important language problems and exert a dragging rather than a stimulating effect on the teaching staff. The difficulty in evaluating foreign medical schools was dramatically illustrated by the fact that the same foreign institution was selected by different hospitals most frequently as the one that over the years has supplied the "best" and the "worst" interns and residents.[3]

The study made no attempt to answer three questions that are of critical importance: whether FMGs fail to meet minimum standards of medical competence for the United States, whether

Table 7. Comparative scores obtained by FMGs and USMGs on the 15 individual questions (higher number equals lower competence)

Question	Paired USMGs		Paired FMGs		Unpaired FMGs	
	Mean	S.D.	Mean	S.D.	Mean	S.D.
Acclimatization	1.4788	0.7352	1.8795[a]	0.8698	1.6923	0.7731
Discipline	1.6687	0.8808	1.7229	0.8113	1.6769	0.7668
General duties	1.6182	0.7424	2.0909[a]	0.9133	2.0000[b]	0.9446
History taking	1.5855	0.6534	2.1523[a]	0.8593	2.0806[b]	0.8386
Physical examanations	1.6463	0.6368	2.0959[a]	0.8385	2.0650[b]	0.7623
Basic medical sciences	1.7229	0.6910	2.4634[a]	0.9133	2.3846[b]	0.8538
Doctor-patient relation	1.4967	0.6893	1.9733[a]	0.8402	1.9449[b]	0.8631
Doctor-staff relation	1.6084	0.8197	1.8072	1.8208	1.8217[b]	0.8667
Personal relations	1.5482	0.8033	1.7530	0.7872	1.7984[b]	0.8201
Libraries	1.9030	0.7154	2.1779[a]	0.8787	2.1085	0.9170
Supervision	1.6988	0.7798	2.2061[a]	0.9045	2.1318[b]	0.9349
Learning processes	1.6325	0.7222	2.0783[a]	0.9248	1.9385[b]	0.8571
The teaching staff and the house staff	1.8253	0.8212	2.4000[a]	0.9957	2.3462[b]	0.9900
Independent learning	1.7108	0.7034	2.2289[a]	0.9547	2.0853[b]	0.9320
Potential for medical practice	1.5951	0.7960	2.2209[a]	0.9909	2.1846[b]	0.9264

Source: J. Med. Educ., 43 (1968), 709. Used by permission of the Journal of Medical Education.

[a]Significant difference of paired FMGs from paired USMGs at .01 level of significance, using t.

[b]Significant difference of unpaired FMGs from paired USMGs at .01 level of significance, using t.

they provide minimally adequate medical care in and out of the hospitals in this country; and whether they are prepared for the health care needs of their own people. Rather, it extended the accepted practice in the United States of evaluating student performance through the observations of their supervisors and mentors. It did not conclude that FMGs are professionally incompetent; it did establish the fact that they represent a level of competence significantly lower than the USMGs in the same program of graduate education.

In their studies of FMGs Halberstam and Dacso [4] had somewhat different terms of reference but reached similar conclusions. They were concerned with FMG residents in affiliated hospitals and in selected specialties. Their inquiries were oriented toward certain personality characteristics, such as motivation, and training experiences, which were evaluated by FMGs themselves and by peer USMGs. Their findings agreed with those of our study summarized above, showing that FMGs are absorbed into hospitals without any noticeable modification of training programs made in recognition of the FMG's deficiencies. Halberstam and Dacso also found evidence of FMG dissatisfaction with this unrealistic system of training.

A particularly interesting aspect of their study was the FMGs' self-evaluation of their competence compared with the evaluations made by the USMGs. The FMGs agreed with their supervisors and their colleagues in rating the USMGs above themselves; none rated themselves as "much better" than the USMGs, half conceded the USMGs did work of higher quality, and 72 percent admitted to their own inferior knowledge of basic medical sciences. The supervisors of both groups stated that the need for considerable or constant supervision occurred six times as frequently among FMGs as among USMGs.

EXPERIENCE WITH EXAMINATIONS

As indicated earlier, FMGs are allowed to take the ECFMG examination with no requirements other than graduation from a medical school listed in the WHO *Directory*, that is, without any discrimination regarding country of origin or quality of undergraduate medical education. The questions chosen for the examination are designed to determine the applicant's suitability for internship in an approved hospital in the United States and are not intended to serve any other purpose. The ECFMG regularly publishes the results of the examination and provides confidential reports to individual schools.

For several years the ECFMG has carefully chosen questions from among those already used by the National Board of Medical Examiners for testing graduates of United States and Canadian medical schools. This arrangement makes possible a direct comparison between the results achieved on the same questions by USMGs and FMGs, although more difficult questions have been specifically eliminated by the ECFMG for the latter group.

The chapter on the ECFMG summarizes fully its experience over the last several years. There is a striking difference between the predictable initial failure rate (2 percent) of the USMGs and the actual failures (60 percent) of the FMGs who responded to the same questions. Furthermore, the scores of the FMGs who did pass were heavily concentrated around the minimal passing mark, so that an increase of the passing level to 80 percent rather than the present 75 percent could eliminate half of those who now pass. Table 8 illustrates this point quite strikingly.

The disadvantages of using state board examinations as criteria of medical skills have already been discussed. The examinations are variable in their severity; both FMGs and USMGs range from a relatively high to a virtually zero failure rate on them. The boards also have some advantages for analysis in this review, not the least of which is the very complete annual reporting in the annual State Board issue of the *Journal of the American Medical Association*. Aside from the full documentation available, the state board examinations are taken by FMGs who have almost all previously passed the ECFMG and

Table 8. Percentage distribution of scores on the ECFMG examination

| Range of Scores | Actual distribution of ECFMG candidates | | Expected distribution of U. S. medical students | |
	March 24, 1965	Sept. 15, 1965	March 24, 1965	Sept. 15, 1965
90% or higher	0.09	0.02	4.63	4.53
85% - 89%	2.94	2.62	29.34	28.77
80% - 84%	9.36	8.85	46.28	45.98
74% - 79%	29.98	30.33	18.87	19.40
70% - 73%	22.55	30.47	0.81	0.91
65% - 69%	19.64	20.48	0	0
60% - 64%	9.86	6.54	0	0
below 60%	5.55	0.62	0	0

Source: ECFMG *Annual Report,* 1966, p. 11. Used by permission of the ECFMG.

subsequently have had several years of graduate medical education. Table 9 demonstrates the consistency in the over-all FMG performance on state board examinations over the last 31 years.

In 1966 National Board endorsement accounted for the majority (5609) of newly licensed USMGs, and 11,667 more were licensed by reciprocity. Only 58 FMGs were licensed by endorsement or reciprocity, and the remaining 1352 passed state examinations. This was a characteristic year. The failure rate on all state boards was 38.1 percent for FMGs and 4.2 percent for USMGs. Since 1935 the FMG failure rates have been as high as 59.2 percent (in 1941) and as low as 29 percent (in 1961), with a 31 year average (1935 to 1966) of 40.2 percent. The performance from state to state varies widely; 363 FMGs had a failure rate of 73.6 percent in Illinois in 1966 (compared with 42.4 percent for USMGs), whereas in Michigan the failure rate for 105 FMGs was zero.

PROFESSIONAL QUALITIES

The performance of FMGs on State Board Examinations in four states in 1966 illustrates the ways in which a concentration of applicants applying for licensure in certain states affects national statistics.[5] The four states, Illinois, Maryland, New York, and Virginia, represented 73 percent of all State Board failures by FMGs in 1966. The requirements for medical licensure of FMGs in the four states is as follows: all require internship, and Maryland, New York, and Virginia also require ECFMG certification; Maryland also requires 3 years of hospital service in the United States, New York requires 1 to 2 years of such experience, and Virginia demands 2 years of accredited hospital training. In 1966 a total of 3691 FMGs took State Board examinations in the United States; 2281 passed the examinations, and 1410 or 38.2 percent failed. Of the 3691 FMGs taking the tests, 1960 were in the four states cited above; 925 of them passed, while 1053 or 53 percent failed.

Foreign medical graduates do not necessarily elect to take the examinations that have a reputation for being easy. As Table 10 shows, of the 3691 who tried to become licensed in 1966, 2409 (65 percent) took the examinations in eight states where their failure rate was 50 percent compared with the USMG failure rate of 10 percent in those same states. As expected, in those states where the USMG failure rate is the highest, the failure rate of FMGs is proportionally higher. In New York the majority of USMGs are licensed by National Board endorsement, so that the state examination is almost exclusively for FMGs, who, in 1965 and 1966 had failure rates of 53 percent and 51 percent respectively.[6]

IMPLICATIONS FOR HEALTH CARE

In spite of all their limitations, the data summarized in this chapter are impressive. Considering the total lack of evidence to the contrary, we must conclude that FMGs have a lower level of professional competence than United States medical graduates initially, when they take the ECFMG examination, during

55

Table 9. Physicians examined by State Medical Boards on the basis of credentials obtained in countries other than the United States and Canada, 1935-1966

Year	Number examined	Number passed	Percent failed
1935	437	303	30.7
1936	568	382	35.0
1937	920	637	30.8
1938	1,164	716	38.5
1939	1,691	839	50.4
1940	2,088	948	54.7
1941	1,717	698	59.2
1942	1,630	890	45.4
1943	1,031	518	49.8
1944	691	325	53.0
1945	475	209	56.0
1946	495	221	55.3
1947	601	283	52.9
1948	639	311	51.3
1949	737	319	56.7
1950	799	359	55.0
1951	1,006	524	47.9
1952	1,208	648	46.3
1953	1,463	796	46.3
1954	1,642	943	42.6
1955	1,771	1,042	41.4
1956	1,783	1,012	43.2
1957	2,299	1,345	41.5
1958	2,567	1,518	40.9
1959	2,766	1,870	32.4
1960	2,864	2,013	29.7
1961	2,683	1,890	29.0
1962	2,960	1,980	33.1
1963	2,781	1,861	33.1
1964	3,246	2,215	31.8
1965	3,011	2,043	32.1
1966	3,691	2,281	38.1
Total	53,444	31,939	40.2

Source: *JAMA, 200* (1967), 1071. Used by permission of the *Journal of the American Medical Association*.

Table 10. FMG and USMG performance on State Boards in 8 selected states, 1966

State	Total FMGs (2409)			Total USMGs (602)		
	Number passed	Failed		Number passed	Failed	
		Number	Percent		Number	Percent
Connecticut	48	41	46.1	7	0	0
Illinois	96	267	73.6	19	14	42.4
Indiana	83	41	33.1	179	1	.5
Maine	58	43	42.6	1	0	0
Maryland	175	93	34.7	147	11	6.9
New Jersey	88	47	34.8	11	0	0
New York	426	447	51.2	20	11	35.5
Virginia	228	228	50.0	157	24	13.2
Total:	1,202	1,207	50.1[a]	541	61	10.1[b]

Source: JAMA, 200 (1967), 1107-1117. Used by permission of the Journal of the American Medical Association.

[a]National Average for FMGs: 38.2 percent.
[b]National Average for USMGs: 4.2 percent.

their period of graduate medical education in this country, and finally at the time that they take state board examinations. No direct documentation can be made of the competence of the approximately 30,000 FMGs who have previously completed their years of training and have remained in the United States.[7] Neither are there any data regarding the actual results of health care provided by FMGs in the United States. This is an issue well worth studying.

CHAPTER IV   Foreign Medical Graduates

and United States Immigration Policies

And when statesmen or others worry him too much, then he should leave with his possessions . . . With a firm and steadfast mind one should hold under all conditions that everywhere the earth is below and the sky above, and to the energetic man, every region is his fatherland. — Tycho Brahe, 1597 [1]

Ours is a world of quickening movement, characterized by constantly shifting populations. Mobility has become a way of life and to change home or country is for many a commonplace event. The ability to travel almost anywhere at great speed and relatively low cost has become an inextricable part of the struggle for success, advancement, and understanding in our society. At society's most frenzied level is the Jet Set who live and play on several continents; at its more traditional level are the nomadic tribes who follow the seasons in order to survive. Since the Serpent became Adam's travel agent, men have wandered in search of many things — adventure, El Dorado, freedom, peace, education. The histories of many nations have been written by their immigrants, whether they came as invading conquerors or in peace, and the fabrics of many societies have been woven by outsiders who immigrated, bringing with them their cultures and their talents.

It is still uncertain to what extent the spread of various cul-

59

tures was due to trade and commerce, or to what extent it involved the wholesale movement of peoples. Certainly the Teutons were noted for their movements *en masse*, and during the Bronze Age and the Iron Age great migrations established the spread of Indo-European languages over the continent of Europe. Greek- and Illyrian-speaking people came down through the Balkans to Greece; Italic-speaking people moved into Italy; Swedes populated Russia; Celts traveled west through central and northern Europe into France and Great Britain. Later Slavic and Teutonic groups followed the same routes. Much later in history the British, French, Dutch, and Spanish spread out from their lands into the New World. They came first as conquerors but remained permanently.

The United States is a nation whose genius and very existence are derived from immigrants. Its astonishing history has been shaped by those who left their native lands and emigrated to North America for a myriad of reasons. Some were paupers, some aristocrats; some were artisans and adventure seekers, others refugees from oppression and men who were dedicated to an ideal which they wanted to pursue in a new land. America is the child of Britain and a descendant of Europe, but her roots also trace back to Greece and Rome and Palestine. No other nation in the history of the world that has been so nurtured by immigration has succeeded as has the United States. In the process, almost every immigrant has become completely immersed in the new life here; and while being assimilated into American society he has managed to maintain some of his past, to contribute some of the culture he brought with him. As Santayana put it, "to be an American is of itself almost a moral condition, an education and a career."

Since the Second World War, the tides of worldwide immigration have again begun to swell. Unlike many of the invasions of past history, most of these invasions have been peaceful. The same forces that propelled the movements of peoples in the past are still at work today. Economic, social, and political conditions throughout the world are still conducive to migration. The forces of "push" and "pull," the great disparities between the rich nations and the poor, exercise a tremendous influence on today's immigration patterns. Italian and Greek laborers have helped reconstruct modern Germany and have supplied the muscle power for her *Wirtschaftswunder*. Indians, Pakistanis, and West Indians have given Great Britain many of her skilled and unskilled workers. Latin American domestic help has partly replenished the dwindling supply in the United States. European refugees have provided Latin America with a vital source of technicians, professionals, and artisans. American citizens, like the ancient Romans, have become ubiquitous in their presence throughout the world as advisors, technicians, students, and tourists.

In a few short years the very fact of mobility has caused borders to open wide. A pass is all that is required to go from one to another of the European Common Market countries. Goods and people flow readily in the free world, and one nation's knowledge is generally another's instant gain. Mass communication and vast transportation facilities make for easy access to borders and to ideas. In a very real sense, then, restrictive immigration policies, at least in the free-world countries, are anachronistic.

The first step in the United States' liberalization of its immigration policies occurred in 1962, when persons with special education and skills were allowed to enter the country without regard to national quotas if they had made application for a Permanent Resident visa prior to April 1, 1962. In 1965 the United States further revised its immigration laws, and with the revisions came a new variation on an old theme. In effect, past prejudices were abolished insofar as restrictive quotas on immigration into the United States were concerned; this country also served notice to the world that it had long taken their tired

61

and poor and now preferred to take their talented. This thought is humorously summed up in a paraphrasing of the inscription on the Statue of Liberty:

> "Give me your tired, your poor,
> Your huddled masses yearning to breathe free,
> The wretched refuse of your teeming shore.
> Send these, the homeless, tempest-tossed to me.
> I lift my lamp beside the golden door."

> "Send me your trained, your skilled,
> Your eager students straining for degrees,
> The cultured cream of all your learned scores.
> Send these, the brainy masters, Ph.D.'s.
> We're courting class along these golden shores." [2]

The Immigration Act of 1952 (McCarran-Walter Act) was amended by Congress on October 3, 1965. The new act, latest in a long series of immigration laws enacted by Congress since the beginning of the 19th century, did not promulgate a new policy, for its concept dated back to earlier decades. The major features of the new law are: the immediate elimination of the Asia–Pacific Triangle provisions and, after a two-and-a-half-year transition period, the abolition of the national origins quota system. An annual ceiling of 170,000 was established on quota immigration with a limitation of not more than 20,000 numbers to be made available to natives of any single foreign state. Since July 1, 1968 quota numbers have been distributed on a first-come, first-served basis within the preference and nonpreference categories and within the 170,000 over-all limitation and 20,000 limit per foreign state. Since that same date, and for the first time in United States immigration history, an annual ceiling of 120,000 has been placed on immigration from the Western Hemisphere.

The legislation established the following new preference categories:

Classes	Description
First Preference:	Unmarried sons and daughters of United States citizens
Second Preference:	Spouses and unmarried sons and daughters of aliens lawfully admitted for permanent residence
Third Preference:	Members of the professions or persons of exceptional ability in the sciences or arts
Fourth Preference:	Married sons or daughters of United States citizens
Fifth Preference:	Brothers or sisters of United States citizens
Sixth Preference:	Skilled or unskilled workers in short supply
Seventh Preference:	Refugees

An important feature of the new Act is that it requires an individual determination by the Secretary of Labor in all cases of third- and sixth-preference and nonpreference-category immigrants. The Secretary of Labor must find in such cases "(a) there are not sufficient workers in the United States who are able, willing, qualified and available at the time of application for a visa and admission to the United States and at the place to which the alien is destined to perform such skilled or unskilled labor, and (b) the employment of such aliens will not adversely affect the wages and working conditions of the workers in the United States similarly employed." [3]

Third- and sixth-preference petitions are not to be approved without the required Labor Certification unless the alien is to be employed in a field found by the Department of Labor to have a shortage of qualified persons in the country. In such cases it is not necessary to make an individual application for the certification. This is the crucial point to understand when considering the subject of immigration of FMGs into the country. It is also the pivotal point of the Labor Department's ruling in December 1965 that, since there is a shortage of doctors in this country, fully licensed physicians from abroad may petition for a Permanent Resident visa without applying for Labor Department clearance.[4] The impact of this decision can have far-reaching effects.

BACKGROUND: UNITED STATES IMMIGRATION LAWS

The first Immigration Act in the United States, passed in 1819, required all captains of vessels entering United States ports to give an account of their passengers to port authorities. From 1820 until the end of the century, northern European immigration to the United States predominated. In the late nineteenth century and early part of the twentieth century Italians, Russians, and Austro-Hungarians contributed heavily to American immigration. One can almost reconstruct the upheavals in Europe during this period in the waves of immigration to the United States. During the middle years of the nineteenth century there was a large influx of peoples of Asiatic origin. In 1834, in response to the heavy immigration, a political party was founded in Philadelphia which called itself the American Republican Party and pledged to obtain a new immigration law that would require a residence of 21 years before eligibility for citizenship. The party failed, but agitation to stop immigration from unpopular areas continued. By 1880 the Congress was prepared to put an end to immigration from the Orient and passed the first of several "Chinese Exclusion Acts" and made a "gentlemen's" (exclusion) agreement with Japan. It is interesting to note that the United States was several decades ahead of such countries as Australia and South Africa, which also passed restrictive immigration acts to exclude Orientals from their countries. In 1902 the Australians passed their exclusion act, and in 1913 South Africa aimed its legislation at the Indians.

During the period immediately preceding World War I and

during the war itself, immigration to the United States decreased considerably. After the war new waves of immigrants began arriving, causing the Congress to pass America's first Quota Act on May 19, 1921. Quotas were based on the Census of 1920 (national origins of white persons) and established on a world-wide basis. Nonetheless, until 1930 almost 200,000 immigrants entered the United States each year. This rate of immigration was possible even though Congress added a visa system in 1924 that made a prospective immigrant establish his right to come in under his country's quota, prove his good character, his lack of either a communist or anarchist affiliation, and the unlikelihood of his becoming a public charge. In fact, in theory, and in practice this complicated system of visas and quotas implemented America's preference for northern European immigrants.

In the depression years immigration dropped as the United States strictly enforced the "public charge" clause of the 1921 Act. In addition, economic conditions, both worldwide and within this country, were not propitious for emigration. From 1936 until 1941 annual immigration ranged between 21,000 and 56,000 persons, including many who were political refugees from European tyranny. During the war years immigration remained slight, but since World War II it has increased constantly. The quota has never been oversubscribed, however, although annual immigration has averaged 100,000 for the past ten years.

IMMIGRATION POLICIES AND FOREIGN STUDENTS

In 1936 the United States Government officially launched its program of promoting better understanding through encouraging mutual exchanges among students. As a part of its Good Neighbor Policy the United States signed the Convention of Buenos Aires in 1936, which contained articles encouraging hemispheric student exchanges. This Convention was renegotiated in Caracas in 1954 and remains in effect today.

FOREIGN MEDICAL GRADUATES

With the passage of the Fulbright Act of 1946, the United States began in earnest its policy of promoting international good will and understanding through students. This international program for educational and cultural exchange of the Department of State was extended in 1948 by the Smith-Mundt Act, which authorized the annual appropriation of United States funds to be used jointly with certain foreign currencies designated for educational purposes. In 1961 these programs were further refined, extended, and supported by the Mutual Educational and Cultural Exchange Act (Fulbright-Hays Act).

The exchange programs have been eminently successful. Their basic purpose, to promote better understanding among participating nations, has been one of the cornerstones of postwar American foreign policy and has achieved widespread support both within the United States and abroad. It is becoming increasingly apparent, however, that many foreign students are beginning to use the Exchange Visitors' Program as an avenue for immigration to the United States. This is possible even though a foreign student with an Exchange Visitor's visa (type J) who has completed his studies in this country is committed to return to his home country, or go to a third country, for a minimum period of two years before he can even apply for a Permanent Resident visa.

A *Progress Report* published by the State Department on March 8, 1966 reported that only 3 percent of all exchange visitors had remained in the United States. In another study covering the period 1962 to 1964 the State Department reported that 90,350 exchange visitors arrived in the United States and that 1528 (1.6 percent) of these ultimately adjusted their status to become permanent residents.[5] Data continue to be conflicting in this area. For example, estimates vary from Professor Grubel's thesis that approximately 10 percent of the exchange visitors remain permanently in the United States to a recent statement in Lausanne that 90 percent of the Asian students remain in this country after completing their studies.[6] No one knows how many persons fulfill the requirement for two-year residency abroad and subsequently return to the United States. As will be discussed later, it should be possible to obtain full data on the number of aliens who annually depart from the United States.

The Mutual Educational and Cultural Exchange Act (Public Law 87–256), enacted on September 21, 1961, stipulates that the Attorney General "may waive the requirement of the two-year foreign residency abroad in the case of any alien whose admission to the United States is found by the Attorney General to be in the public interest." The Department of State has received such a large number of applications for waiver of the two-year residence requirement that it has established an Exchange Visitor's Waiver Review Board. The Board is served by two Executive Secretaries, one of whom receives applications for waivers by Exchange Visitors in the health and biomedical fields alone. The other receives applications from all fields other than health. It is significant that one of the Secretaries devotes full time to the medical field, and the most recent publication from the State Department's Bureau of Cultural and Social Affairs presents ample data for explaining this phenomenon. In fiscal year 1962, for example, 3970 physicians and surgeons entered the United States as Exchange Visitors. Four years later 755 of these physicians and surgeons were known to have received waivers from the Immigration and Naturalization Service (INS), which had granted a total of only 1701 waivers to Exchange Visitors in all fields.[7]

SUMMARY OF VISA CLASSIFICATIONS

At this point it would be well to review briefly the types of visas which are issued for entry into the United States. There are many types of visas, which cover the alphabet from "A" through "SE3," but the majority are applicable only in very special circumstances and are fairly rigidly controlled. For instance, it is possible for a student to possess an A visa, but this is applicable only to persons (including family members) entitled to diplomatic status. Another type is the H visa, which is reserved for various classes of "aliens of distinguished merit and ability." Usually a professor qualifies in this category; a cabaret singer will also qualify. Other examples are: NATO visa, for personnel representing NATO countries; SE-1 visa, for alien employees of the United States government abroad; SD-1 visa, for ministers of religion; and so on.

There are basically two types of visa arrangements by which FMGs enter the United States. In order to understand clearly the distinctions that are made by the United States consular officers abroad before they issue a visa to an FMG, these two types should be well defined. Their official categories are the J visa and the Permanent Resident visa. The former is classified as "nonimmigrant," and the latter is in the immigration-permanent resident classification.

The granting of a J visa is the responsibility of the United States consular officer abroad. It is his duty to ascertain if an applicant for a J visa meets the qualifications set forth in the Fulbright-Hays Act of 1961 (the Mutual Educational and Cultural Exchange Act). Under a very complex series of arrangements the United States has established a wide range of exchange programs, and nationals of other countries who wish to come to America under one of these programs are granted J visas. Between 1962 and 1964 approximately 90,350 Exchange Visitors came to the United States. Since the beginning of fiscal year 1961, there have been 21,644 foreign medical graduates who have entered the United States with J visas.

The length of stay granted to a holder of a J visa is contingent upon the course of study he intends to pursue. Doctors of medicine are granted J visas for a five-year period. This allows them sufficient time for the completion of both an internship and a residency program and perhaps to become certified as a specialist if they choose to do so. It is also possible to apply for an extension of stay beyond this five-year period.

Before a consular officer grants a J visa to an FMG, he requires a completed DSP/66 form. This form is supplied by a United States hospital which has been approved for an Exchange Visitor Program, and which has subsequently been given a so-called "P" number. The DSP/66 is ultimately surrendered by the FMG at his port of entry into the United States and in its place an INS Form 1–94 is inserted in his passport which indicates his visa type, date of entry, duration of visa period, and place of entry into the country.[8]

At the time of application for a J visa the applicant formally declares, by signing document Forms DSP/37 and DSP/66, that he understands the nature of his entry into the United States, the limitations on his stay, and the two-year residency abroad requirement. These are the main features of the J visa, and they are amplified and explained to applicants by the United States consular officers.

Persons admitted as Permanent Residents into the United States may accept employment and may apply for citizenship, although they have no obligation to do so. There are many different classes of preference categories for the issuance of immigrant visas. The usual categories under which FMGs qualify are third and sixth preference — a professional of exceptional ability and a person whose skills are in short supply in this country.

Assuming that an FMG qualifies under the third or sixth preference categories, he may request a Permanent Resident visa from the consular officer in his country. At that time he must present his birth certificate, his police record and his military record, submit to a medical examination, pay a fee for the visa ($25), and show evidence that he is not likely to become a public charge in the United States. It is not necessary for an FMG to have an approved petition from the Department

69

of Labor. A male applicant who is over 18 years of age and born on or after September 15, 1925 must submit a statement indicating his understanding of the fact that he has a legal obligation to register for military service with a local board of the Selective Service System within six months of the date on which he enters the United States.

In fiscal year 1966, there were 2552 FMGs who entered the United States with Permanent Resident visas, and in fiscal year 1967 the number increased to 3336, representing a 30 percent increase in the first year of operation for the new immigration law. These FMGs are officially considered immigrants to the United States and have all the rights and privileges, responsibilities, and duties which attend that status. They are, quite obviously, in a category that is clearly distinct from Exchange Visitors.

THE NEW IMMIGRANT

The impact of the new immigration policies has not yet been felt in the United States; but, while no patterns have been clearly established, certain trends are already discernible. For example, after the liberalization began in 1962 there was a dramatic rise in immigration from Asia in 1963 and 1964.[9] One of the basic tenets of the Act, however, appears to be to make immigration more selective through measures which favor individuals with high levels of training. This is true even though another basic purpose of the Act is to make immigration policies more equitable and to liberalize quota restrictions. Since it abandons America's long-established national-origins basis of quota allocations for immigration, it also encourages immigration from the developing regions of the world.[10] Since July 1, 1968, immigrants have been admitted on the basis of the order in which they apply for visas, regardless of their country of birth. Another stipulation of the Act is that from fiscal year 1969 onward, non-Western Hemisphere countries will be limited to a global quota of 170,000, and a Western Hemisphere quota of 120,000 has been set for the first time. An annual quota of 17,000 was established for professional and highly skilled persons in third and sixth preference categories. In June 1966, there were 3000 professional and skilled workers waiting to have their Permanent Resident visas processed. By June 1967, this figure had risen to 8400.[11] These 11,000 persons were reflected in the actual immigration figures for fiscal years 1967 and 1968, and it is certain that thousands of FMGs were among them.

THE FOREIGN MEDICAL GRADUATE AND AMERICA'S NEW OPEN-DOOR POLICY

Nowhere has the impact of foreign students in recent years been more pronounced than in the field of medicine. It should be made quite clear at this point that FMGs represent a special situation, for while the large majority of them come to the United States with Exchange Visitors visas (J), they are far more than students. They have received their education abroad and have come to this country for advanced training. They also supply skills and services as they train. They are paid for these services and are, therefore, a part of the United States labor market. They assume duties which include caring for United States citizens and are, consequently, entrusted with heavy responsibilities.

Inadvertently, perhaps, the new Immigration Act favors physicians. This is partially due to America's physician shortage, but also it is quite apparent that a physician is the prototype envisaged in the new Act's third and sixth preference categories. The FMG's acceptability is further enhanced by the Department of Labor's ruling that there is a shortage of physicians in the United States and, therefore, no Labor Department clearance is necessary prior to the issuance of a Permanent Resident visa for a physician. An alien physician may send his petition for a

71

Permanent Resident visa (Form 1–140) directly to the INS. Other categories of petitioners for such visas must first be approved by the Department of Labor (Form 575A).

If an alien physician's supporting documents are in order, INS adjudicates the alien clearance, and the United States consular officer abroad is notified that he may issue a Permanent Resident visa when the other papers are certified. Under the terms of the Labor Department's definition of a physician, the alien physician must show evidence with supporting documents that (1) he is a graduate of a United States medical school, or (2) he is a graduate of a foreign medical school and has passed the ECFMG examination, or (3) that he is a graduate of a foreign medical school and has a full, unrestricted license to practice medicine and two years' gainful employment in his profession. In support of the Labor Department, the State Department has notified its consulates abroad (Airgrams in 1963, 1965, and 1966) that consular officers should stress the need for ECFMG certification but that a full, unrestricted license to practice medicine and two years' gainful employment may be accepted in lieu of the ECFMG certification. For the purposes of the INS it is the intention of the FMG that is the main consideration. If the alien petitions for a Permanent Resident visa with the intent to practice medicine, this satisfies INS requirements.

Point 3 of the Labor Department's ruling is inconsistent with existing policies in effect in all states in this country. The Labor Department, the State Department, and the INS permit physicians without ECFMG certification to enter the country with Permanent Resident visas and with the intent to practice their profession. In point of fact, they cannot at the time of entry legally practice medicine.

U.S. policy has been to accept, if not encourage, the immigration of physicians into this country even at the expense of admitting those whose only qualifications are derived from the

72

fact that they have been in practice for two years in some other country. That we accept them, of course, does not mean that they can automatically become practitioners in this country. But acceptance can also lead to disenchantment, false hopes, or illegal practice. Whichever of these may occur, the fact is that we are responsible for these physicians and so too is the American public.

It is increasingly obvious that more and more FMGs are arriving in the United States every year, that more are coming with Permanent Resident visas, that more waivers are being granted to those with J visas, and that the upward trend will continue. Table 11 reflects the trend over the past decade.

Table 11. Number of FMGs entering the United States on Permanent Resident Visas, 1957-1967

Year	No.
1957	1990
1958	1934
1963	2093
1964	2249
1965	2012
1966	2552
1967	3336

Source: United States Department of Justice, Immigration and Naturalization Service

That an FMG possesses a Permanent Resident visa does not preclude his ultimate return to his home country; neither does it necessarily mean that he will become a naturalized United States citizen. However, many of these FMGs will remain here permanently if past history is any guide, and they will continue to swell the ranks of the new licentiates every year. As Table 12 indicates, the number of FMGs who represent new additions to the medical profession is increasing each year.

Table 12. FMGs representing new additions to the medical
profession, selected years, 1950-1965

Year	Number	Percent of total additions
1950	308	5.1
1959	1626	19.7
1960-1965	average of 1300	17.0

Source: *JAMA*, *200* (1967), 1072. Used by permission of the *Journal of
the American Medical Association*.

Perhaps the most important point in this discussion of the
immigration of foreign physicians is the fact that the majority
who do elect to remain here permanently are from the developing areas of the world. Since immigration has been restrictive
for these persons in the past, most have been coming on Exchange Visitor visas. Now that immigration is open to them,
they will almost certainly be using Permanent Resident visas.
Appendix Table B9 summarizes in rank order the countries of
origin of FMGs in graduate programs as of December 31, 1966.
Particularly significant is the fact that since December 31, 1965,
Korea rose from 11th place to 3d place and Thailand moved
from 13th to 5th. The four nations whose trainees increased
over 100 each in the past year (Philippines, Korea, India,
Thailand) are all in Asia. Data that are available indicate that
over 80 percent of the FMGs who receive waivers are from the
less developed countries.[12] We have already seen that 45 percent of all waivers are given to physicians and surgeons; and
that 17 percent of all the Exchange Visitor physicians are given
waivers and that of these the overwhelming majority are from
countries to which we have long been giving technical assistance.

It is virtually impossible to arrive at a valid economic interpretation of the value to the United States of physician immigration. That at least 8500 FMGs entered the United States in

fiscal year 1967 is a known fact. This is offset, however, by the unknown number of FMGs who left the country during the same year. Responsible officials in the State Department are confident that the large majority of FMGs with J visas remain in the country for their full five years, and FMGs with Permanent Resident visas may stay as long as they choose. It seems likely, owing to these factors, that there are distinct monetary advantages which accrue to the United States by virtue of this large annual influx of foreign-trained physicians. Although the exact dimensions of this gain are difficult to assess, it can be pointed out that to construct one new medical school would cost at least $50 million and that the annual operating costs of a medical school average $3.8 million.[13]

Table 13 indicates the extent to which the United States has become dependent upon foreign physicians since 1960. The data for 1966–67 should be examined separately, for that was the first fiscal year in which the amended Immigration Act was in effect: [14]

Year July 1– June 30	Immi- grants	Exchange Visitors	FMG Total	Graduates U.S. Medi- cal Schools	Ratio FMG: USMG
1966–67	3336	5204	8540	7743	110.3

Until fiscal year 1967 the United States had been importing a substantial number of foreign physicians, primarily for service in hospitals. The number of FMGs entering the United States each year never exceeded the number of annual graduates from medical schools in this country. In fiscal year 1967, however, the situation changed, and 797 more FMGs than USMGs entered the United States' health care system.

Immigration, as we have seen, is a way of life as old as the history of man. It is also a healthy, vital, and constructive force that contributes to national growth and international understanding. Brain drain is a relatively recent phenomenon which is quickly becoming part and parcel of national immigration

Table 13. Comparison of total number of FMGs admitted to U. S. with numbers of USMGs, 1961-1966

| Year | FMGs | | | USMGs | Ratio |
(July 1-June 30)	Immigrants	Exchange Visitors	Total		FMG:USMG
1961-1962	1,796	3,970	5,767	7,168	80.5
1962-1963	2,093	4,637	6,730	7,264	92.6
1963-1964	2,249	4,518	6,767	7,335	92.3
1964-1965	2,012	4,160	6,172	7,409	83.3
1965-1966	2,552	4,370	6,922	7,574	91.4
Total	10,703	21,655	32,358	36,751	88

Source: Data compiled from INS and AAMC statistics.

policy deliberations. Ideally, there should be a clear distinction between the idea of free movement of peoples and national ownership of talent. Unfortunately, immigration and brain drain (or its reverse, "brain gain") complement, indeed feed upon, each other. This subject will be discussed more thoroughly in Chapter V. Thoughtful officials in most countries, particularly the more developed ones, do not wish to impose restrictive immigration policies. Certainly the United States, which for so long imposed harsh national quotas, does not want to revise its Immigration and Nationality Act again. Some of the features of the 1965 revision still have not gone into effect, and there is great reluctance to begin tampering with them at this juncture.

In the pursuit of equality and freedom of movement many inequities will occur. It is extremely difficult to assess the long-range effects of a policy that has had only a short life. Very often a system will take care of itself. Countervailing forces are constantly at work in any mechanism, and this is particularly true where a combination of social, economic, and political forces is involved, as is the case with the complicated immigration structure. There is ample evidence that most responsible United States officials favor readjusting any imbalances created by the new immigration legislation through outside processes and negotiations, but without further amendments to the Act itself. This would, of course, be most desirable.

It remains to be seen, however, whether the United States can meet its health manpower needs from within its own resources, or whether it will continue to use the liberalized immigration policy as a convenient avenue for supplying its needs with trained physicians from abroad.

CHAPTER V   The Foreign Medical Graduate
and the Brain Drain

I am an individual . . . I give my allegiance as a free man to those
agencies most likely to meet my criteria for a meaningful existence.
— An Anonymous British Immigrant to the United States — 1964 [1]

"Brain drain" is a term which time has proved to be more
convenient than descriptive. It implies more than it says and
disguises what should be made more apparent. Nevertheless,
we shall continue to use the term after further agreement on the
kind of shorthand it represents.

A relatively tasteless translation of "brain drain" is "loss of
human capital investments," and a less inclusive term is "migration of talented or highly skilled individuals." A short economic
definition is "rational allocation of scarce resources." For many
who are deeply — and at times emotionally — concerned with
the issues, it is the unwarranted and undesirable loss of urgently
needed, highly educated individuals from poor countries to
more fortunate countries like ours which could get along very
well without them. There is equal concern, however, on the part
of relatively affluent countries like England because they are
losing to the even more affluent Unites States many skilled
people who the British Government thinks should remain at
home.

Our discussion will be confined to health manpower and, for
convenience, will be focused on physicians from developing

countries. Furthermore, we prefer to minimize vaporous philosophizing by stating at the outset that there *is* a significant brain drain that is harmful to countries the United States prefers to help, and in certain ways harmful also to this country. To some extent this condition is based on the authors' moral judgments; it is also based upon known data and inferences drawn from analyzing these data.

We may begin our discussion with the simple postulate that the rich should not prosper at the expense of the poor. Despite the hazards of using physician-to-population ratios it is not difficult to accept the fact that a disease-burdened country which has less than one physician for 5000 people should not lose its physicians to a country that has one for every 700 rather healthy people.

Any country which has invested from very limited resources in the establishment of a medical school deserves to benefit from the individuals who are finally graduated from that most costly of all educational systems. Despite our deep faith in individual freedom and human rights, we are also convinced that anyone who has been educated at the expense of his country has some obligation to serve his own people although he may live more prosperously elsewhere. Certainly it is not for citizens of the United States to encourage the personal ambitions of a foreign physician if those ambitions run counter to the responsibilities he assumed when he entered a medical school created and maintained in the national interest of his homeland.

The foregoing comments would be mere quibbling if the dimensions of physician migration were not so great. The data from the Immigration and Naturalization Service (Table 13 in Chapter IV) are striking, showing that the number of FMGs entering the United States each year almost equals the number of our own medical school graduates. Table 14 compares the same number of FMGs in the United States on December 31, 1966 with the number of physicians in their own countries.

Table 14. Numbers of FMGs in the U. S. compared with numbers of
physicians in their countries of graduation

Country	FMGs in U. S.	Physicians in country of graduation	Physicians graduated annually	Total population of country (thousands)
Bolivia	84	895	–	3,416
Colombia	596	7,453	442	14,447
Dominican Republic	328	2,085	85	3,014
Haiti	174	400	41	3,505
Nicaragua	40	524	22	1,450
Greece	624	10,400	424	8,350
Taiwan	440	6,901	401	12,180
South Korea	1,060	7,100	600	22,944
Philippines	5,056	18,266	1,010	27,088
India	1,833	85,000	3,100	439,073
Thailand	602	3,815	225	22,718
Iran	1,000	7,090	600	22,860

Source: Combination of statistics from AMA data, the WHO Directory of
Medical Schools (1963), and unpublished documents of the Pan American
Health Organization. The AMA data are for December 31, 1966, and the
WHO and PAHO data are one to three years older.

It is revealing to note from Table 14 that the 40 Nicaraguan
physicians in this country approximate the total medical school
output of Nicaragua for two years, and that the 328 physicians
from the Dominican Republic represent their medical school
output for four years. Despite its large physician manpower
supply India can ill afford to send almost 2000 of its medical
graduates to the United States in addition to the very large
number who go to the United Kingdom. Iran and Thailand are
relatively well supplied with physicians, but the United States
has approximately one of their medical graduates for every five
still at home.

If the United States lost 60,000 of its own medical graduates
to other countries, the equivalent of Iran's or Thailand's loss to

this country, for even brief assignments, there would be widespread cries of shock and outrage. If we added to that migration the repatriation of all FMGs now in this country, the total number of physicians remaining would be reduced from 300,000 to 200,000. Even so, we would still have one physician for every 1000 people, an enviable goal for the less developed countries.

Few will disagree with the principles or even the sentiments we are defending, but some will argue that they are naïve. It has been correctly asserted that there is a great difference between the biomedical needs of developing countries and their economic or social readiness to meet those needs. Physicians leave poor countries because they cannot find employment, because there are inadequate facilities for the skills they possess, because there is no support for their research, or because the opportunities for professional advancement are restricted. Not infrequently the health officials in the FMGs' countries agree with the validity of their complaints. Almost one in every four FMGs in the United States is from the Philippines, but the President of the Philippine Medical Association, Dr. Pacifico Marcos, denied that this represented brain drain. He explained that the medical schools in the Philippines graduate far more doctors than the nation can employ in desirable positions, that they will not go where they are most needed, but that there is a shortage of teachers and researchers.[2] On the other hand, Dr. Francisco T. Dalupan, former President of the University of the East, Manila, has said: "To be blunt about it, are not Philippine medical schools, by operation of this exodus, subsidizing American hospitals?"[3]

Those who argue against the evidence of brain drain think, as does Dr. Marcos, that physicians who will accept nothing but an attractive position at home should be allowed to emigrate to the United States where prospects are brighter. But what would happen if the escape hatch were closed? One possibility is that the competition for urban medical practice would force those who would otherwise refuse to go out into rural areas to do so. Another possibility is that the apparent overproduction of medical graduates would be corrected, thus diverting wasted medical funds into support for better community health care. Medical school enrollments could be reduced to sensible numbers, with a corresponding increase in the quality of medical education from which all would benefit.

It is illogical for the United States to absorb the overflow from wasteful systems so effectively that the deficiencies of these systems are neither discovered nor corrected. It is also highly imprudent for us to pass judgment on the ability of any country to use its skilled manpower to carry out its national health plans. On the other hand, we have received many protests from other countries regarding brain drain, but we have received no requests from them to skim off any excess of physicians or nurses because they are not employable or otherwise useful.

Just as the migration of FMGs has blurred the problems in other countries, so it has effectively disguised some of our own shortcomings. Until recently assessments of health manpower resources and predictions of future needs have blandly ignored the fact that we are not self-sufficient, that we maintain our physician-to-population ratios through the importation of FMGs, mostly from developing countries. In some sections of the country we have become so dependent on FMGs that there are serious doubts that we could meet patient needs without them.[4]

There is an ironic aspect of the medical brain drain problem which has not gone unnoticed and which is highly controversial. Like the phrase "brain drain" itself, this problem has many faces. It is called either "brain drain in reverse" or reverse foreign assistance. Those who support the thesis that the United States is the principal beneficiary from the brain drain contend that we have become a debtor nation regardless of our intentions. During the years in which our foreign aid programs for health have declined there has been a rapid increase in our utilization of physicians from the developing countries of the world. Professor Titmuss has estimated that the United States has saved $4 billion since 1949 with the importation of 100,000 skilled persons, and he stated that recruiting from United States hospitals is constantly increasing, the number of advertisements for health personnel in British medical journals having risen from 134 in 1951 to over 4000 in 1965.[5]

The British have estimated that it takes $21,000 to train a physician in Great Britain and that they lose between 300 and 350 doctors to the United States each year. At the same time Great Britain gains Commonwealth physicians, and 44 percent of Britain's junior medical staff on the government-controlled National Health Service is foreign, primarily Indian and Pakistani. The same general situation prevails in Canada. From 1950 to 1963, some 9800 professional and skilled workers emigrated to the United States from Canada. During the same period, around 26,000 immigrated into Canada.[6]

Some aspects of this balance of trade in skills favorable to the United States are more apparent than real. Thousands of FMGs have returned to their own countries, some to assume major responsibilities in health care systems or in teaching programs, with obvious benefits accruing from their experiences in the United States. Unfortunately, we do not know how many are repatriated, but we do know that virtually all who were government-sponsored have gone home again. For their countries this is a clear gain.

Furthermore, the very nature of graduate medical education in United States hospitals requires involvement of the trainee in direct patient care, that is, in the provision of a valuable and necessary service. It is inevitable that this be thought of as a contribution by the FMG (and his country) to the welfare of an American community. Indeed, if his time is spent primarily or wholly in service with inadequate supervision or teaching, it is largely a one-way contribution rather than an exchange, with net effects that are undesirable for all. Where the internship or residency program is well managed, the FMG and the hospital will both gain; furthermore, the FMG is well paid, with consequent benefits to himself and his dependents. No one has attempted the calculation, but the foreign exchange advantages to developing countries through this arrangement must also be considerable.

Perhaps the weightiest but least measurable factor is the professional character of the FMG's training experiences in the United States. As noted before, hospitals that employ FMGs solely to meet their own service needs are guilty of exploiting not only our immigration procedures but also the unfortunate disparities that exist between our nation and many others. Whether these interns and residents remain here permanently or go back home, the quality of health care may suffer.

A more elusive but equally worrisome issue is the relevance of graduate training in the United States to the needs of the countries to which the FMGs are destined to return. Here the term brain drain may very well be most appropriate. Our advanced, highly sophisticated hospital practices are very alluring, and establish for young physicians a set of standards that they in turn sincerely wish to maintain. We no longer see in our hospitals the diseases that abound in Asia or Africa; instead, we concentrate on such challenging problems as the replacement of heart valves, organ transplants, and the better uses of radioisotopes. The more proficient the FMG the more he will wish to continue with what he has come to accept as the epitome of good medical practice. With rare exceptions he must abandon much of what he has learned so painfully when he goes back to his country of origin. Indeed, he may find that he is not at all proficient in the management of the very diseases he saw in the United States, because he no longer has the personnel and facilities on which he depended while in this country. These circumstances have led to widespread disaffection among recently repatriated physicians, many of whom spend the next several years arranging to return to the United States. There is no need to discuss the violation of educational principles involved in programs that teach inapplicable skills, but it is important to learn more about how frequently this occurs. Knowledge gained by FMGs in this country can be adapted to the markedly different needs of another country, but the likelihood of consistent success is remote. This kind of brain drain may very well be the most damaging. It requires very careful evaluation, and it also requires the cooperation of all countries that will face the situation objectively and without hysteria.

In this and preceding chapters we have not discussed all of the many factors that affect brain drain, but only those that are relevant to the migration of physicians. We have made no attempt to distinguish between the needs of countries that are in vastly different stages of socioeconomic development. For the sake of precision we would prefer not to lump together, for example, the manpower needs of Iran or Taiwan with those of Somalia or Mali. In reality, however, the differences are not very meaningful, for those countries with the slimmest resources suffer less brain drain only in a numerical sense. The losses are equally painful.

We have also attempted to maintain a reasonable degree of objectivity, using dependable data whenever they are available. The temptation to pervert a review of brain drain into a series of accusations has frequently proved irresistible, especially for those most immediately affected both here and abroad. The most serious fault lies with the whole system that is the subject of this monograph, a system made of many disconnected parts with no focus of responsibility. There have been some transgressions, but in general there is remarkable evidence of widespread and enthusiastic efforts to achieve the best possible results for all. There has been no lack of good intentions. As is so often the case, however, good intentions have not been enough; on the contrary, they have frequently been the cause for much that has gone wrong. The basic justification for encouraging physician migration seems indisputable: a better education and improved medical skills are assets needed everywhere. This country has been most generous in sharing with others our programs of medical education which are admired throughout the world. The United States has painstakingly removed odious ethnic restrictions and lifted quotas on immigration; voluntary groups have tried diligently to introduce foreign scholars to the American way of life; examination procedures have been designed to make the path easier for aliens who wish to study here; promising individuals have been given encouragement and unique opportunities they would never have received at home; and restrictive licensure regulations have been relaxed to give greater freedom to those who were educated in other countries.

While these and other events were occurring, no one was measuring the results. There seems to have been a benevolent assumption that nobility of purpose leads inevitably to a happy ending. What did happen has now become evident, even with some of the information still lacking. The United States has been siphoning off medical manpower from areas of the world which can least afford such losses, returning to them physicians with inapplicable skills and doubtful professional careers at home. However inadvertent it may have been, we have frustrated the intent of the Exchange Visitor Program so frequently that what was once laudable now often appears harmful, even to our closest friends.

It should surprise no one that the cries of protest have begun. Those most affected, the poor of many countries, are tragically unaware of what has been happening. Those who are aware have become quite vociferous in their criticisms. We should like to join with them in the search for equitable solutions.

CHAPTER VI Some Dilemmas — Some Solutions

This monograph was written to meet the need for a compilation of the pertinent facts related to FMGs in the United States. In a sense, we have done what we intended without this final chapter. Much of what we have found wrong is the result of inattention, of unawareness or indifference toward such major issues as exploitation of alien physicians, inadequate medical education, erosion of the quality of health care at home and abroad, and brain drain. What now seems to be callousness may be only a sign of carelessness. In any case, bad practices that have been attributed to ignorance can no longer be tolerated in the light of such well-established facts as those we have summarized. It is worth noting that our observations are fully consistent with the judgments and impressions of the majority of those who have been close to the problems of the foreign medical graduate. We have tried to verify these judgments and provide evidence that the issues are even larger than has been generally realized.

Nonetheless, it is reasonable for us to make recommendations that seem meritorious. They are proposed in the belief that they may lead to the kinds of improvements that are both desirable and attainable. We prefer to be specific by directing our recommendations to those organizations or agencies that can respond helpfully without an intolerable dislocation of other related policies or practices. We are well aware of the greater advantages of a coordinated series of changes to produce the best possible results, but in the absence of such a laudable arrangement we remain confident that highly beneficial results can follow relatively independent, sensible actions. At the outset we also want to recognize those issues that are related to FMGs but are, for the moment, either insoluble or outside the province of this monograph.

ISSUES AND NON-SOLUTIONS

In our preface we stressed the special characteristics of FMGs that justified the separate attention we proposed to give them. Any recommendations we have made remain within the framework of the subject as we have defined it. We fully recognize the powerful influences of larger forces that affect all migration but, for our purposes, they are outside of the scope of this discussion.

Economic Insolubles. There are disparities between societies that will continue to influence the movements of their people. For example, the United States has a gross national product which is eight times that of Great Britain, and in 1965 this country spent over four times as much on research and development as either Western Europe or Russia (17,500:4300).[1] Thus, both our economic capacities and our investments in biomedical research have created an almost unfillable market for talent. This attraction will persist and, very possibly, will grow even stronger.

Diplomatic Tensions. The diplomatic consequences of the United States' highly favorable economic position are equally troublesome, as can be illustrated by the following incident. On February 13, 1967, the Conservative Party in Great Britain introduced a motion to censure Prime Minister Harold Wilson's Labor Government for having failed to plug the drain of British doctors and scientists away from England and into the United

States. Mr. Quintin Hogg, a member of the Opposition, contended that the United States has been "plundering the educational systems of Western Europe," and that "the American high school system is not sufficiently good to produce high-class graduates on a scale required by American industry, American universities, and the American Government." [2] After a heated debate, the motion was defeated by a vote of 314 to 233.

Our diplomatic relations with the United Kingdom or other countries will not be severed over such an issue, but events like these do put a strain on the friendliest of governments. Premier Kosygin was well aware of this situation when he suggested to the Europeans that they had better put an end to the technological gap by keeping their scientists and skilled personnel at home. [3]

Educational Prestige. Another related force to be recognized is the great reputation of American medical education. It is almost universally accepted as one of the best and most sophisticated in the world. That it may in fact be relatively inferior for the needs of a less developed country does not diminish its appeal for young physicians everywhere who yearn to study in one of our great centers. The present ferment in medicine will not diminish the stature of our institutions; on the contrary, they will continue to look even more intriguing if they become less available to the FMGs.

Despite the problems involved, the United States will and should continue to provide opportunities for physicians from other countries to study in its universities and hospitals. No change in program planning or selection procedures can diminish the importance of those resources for a world in need of ever-increasing numbers of skilled health workers. Inevitably, many who are attracted to the United States will wish to remain permanently, and some will do so.

A countering force can be found in efforts to upgrade the educational systems in other countries, but it is a force that will have little effect on migration for many years since the development process is by nature slowmoving.

Investments in Health. Compounding the difficult task other countries face in retaining their young medical graduates is this country's willingness to provide adequate support for physicians in graduate programs. The salaries we offer interns and residents, often rather low by United States standards, exceed those earned by professors in many of the less developed countries. This practice will not change; salaries here are more likely to rise, whereas the professors of Asia or Latin America will probably remain underpaid. It has been pointed out that one of the reasons why Venezuela has suffered very little brain drain and has received quite a bit of "brain gain" is that the salaries given to scientific and medical personnel are quite high.[4] If this issue can be resolved, it will require fundamental changes which are outside the scope of this review.

Even the shortages of health manpower encourage increased migration. The United States has many more physicians for our population than have all the countries from which FMGs emigrate, and, in contrast to those countries, our biomedical needs are supported by our readiness to purchase health services. Thus, a country that has less than one doctor for every 5000 people may be unable effectively to employ all of the physicians who are available. In the United States, rural medical practice is highly lucrative on a fee-for-service basis; in India, rural life is fairly miserable and offers the physician virtually no private practice and very low salaries. These differences will probably persist and may even widen.

Freedom of Choice. Finally, we recognize the fact that the phenomena we have been describing are in part the manifestations of free societies. We fully subscribe to the philosophy that led to a liberalization of our immigration laws. Those who wish to become citizens of the United States should not be restricted by any artificial barriers that we as a nation of immigrants may impose upon them. It is noteworthy that brain drain to the United States is not a serious issue in countries where governments rigidly control the movements of their subjects, such as those under Communist rule. Just as we must keep open our doors to others, so also must other democratic societies permit freedom of exit for their citizens. In the search for a better life hundreds of thousands will suffer the uncertainties of dislocation for themselves and their families, traveling short or great distances as opportunities beckon them. There is probably more gain than loss in such mobility, and it will continue.

PRINCIPLES AND SOLUTIONS

Whatever is done to solve the problems of FMGs must be predicated on clearly defined goals which govern their education and utilization. We shall exercise the freedom of authorship by stating those goals, supported by the knowledge that they almost surely represent the consensus within the medical profession, educational institutions, and governmental agencies in the United States. The goals follow without further comment:

I. The United States should fulfill its responsibility and capability to meet the health care needs of its citizens entirely from its own resources. This should be done by marked expansion of our own medical school output and without planned dependence on FMGs.

II. Foreign medical graduates who do come to the United States for graduate education should be trained to meet the health care needs of their own countries. They should be educated only in institutions that have programs designed for that purpose rather than in hospitals that have internships and residencies designed solely for our society and our system of health care.

III. Foreign medical graduates who intend to remain in this country permanently should be distinguished from those who plan to return to their countries of origin. The two groups should be selected differently, should meet different professional standards, and should receive different kinds of education.

IV. All physicians who provide health care in the United States should be given equal treatment, regardless of their country of education. There should be no relaxation of requirements for medical licensure or for the assumption of other responsibilities or privileges that would in any way diminish the quality of health services which the physician provides.

V. Immigration laws should remain free of discriminatory ethnic restrictions, either direct or indirect, and should be equally unbiased in the freedom of entry allowed physicians who wish to migrate to the United States. The issuance of visas to physicians on an occupational basis should be consistent with the laws that govern medical practice in the United States rather than those that govern medical practice in the countries of origin.

VI. Records should be maintained and published, in the United States and elsewhere, to make possible effective evaluation of the results of physician migration and to provide the information needed for continued monitoring and modification of the programs associated with their migration.

PROFESSIONAL RESPONSIBILITIES AND ACTIONS

Medical standards and practices in the United States are controlled or dominated by voluntary professional organizations, particularly those that make up the governing body of the Education Council for Foreign Medical Graduates. The most influential forces that affect FMGs are centralized in the hospitals employing them as interns and residents. Through the hospitals' methods of appointment and training they determine selection, qualifications, manner of education, utilization in patient care services, and subsequent career choices of FMGs. Without in any manner altering the regulations of the Immigration and Naturalization Service the voluntary system can bring about striking changes which will rectify many of the present deficiencies.

SOME DILEMMAS — SOME SOLUTIONS

This goal may be achieved by a series of policy decisions to be followed by appropriate modifications in the practices not only of the ECFMG but also of the AMA, the AAMC, and the American Hospital Association (AHA), which are the key trustees of the ECFMG as well as independent bodies. In these policy setting capacities they are the logical organizations through which changes are channeled.

The first policy decision that should be made is to separate those FMGs who are migrating as permanent residents to the United States from those who will be returning to their own countries. It is much simpler, and more appropriate, for this separation to be achieved without attempting to alter the issuance of visas or the rules that govern their use.

The distinction can be readily accompanied through a basic change in the manner of selection and by the use of two kinds of qualifying examinations. Those foreign physicians, whether on Permanent Resident or Exchange Visitor visas, who state their intention of returning to their own countries should be chosen through the cooperation of the governmental bodies or institutions that will employ them when they go home. They should be placed exclusively in United States programs that meet requirements to be defined by the ECFMG or its trustee members, programs that are clearly related to the health needs and professional careers of this select group of FMGs. These FMGs should not be eligible for appointment as interns or residents in programs currently approved by the AMA's Council on Medical Education unless they change their status and follow the procedures described below. Preference should be given to more mature physicians who will subsequently assume important roles in teaching, research, or health care in their own countries. FMGs should not be given responsibilities for patient care in this country except as a part of their education, and then only under close supervision. Rather, they should be given full opportunities for supplementary education in the scientific disciplines or organizational aspects of medicine that will be of

93

value to them. The ECFMG examination which they take prior to entering a program in the United States should be used primarily for placement. Greater dependence should be placed on the selection process used by their home institutions, which can better determine the individual's qualifications for the duties he will be asked to perform on his return.

There is ample precedent for this kind of restricted, explicitly goal-related plan. For many years international agencies, including the United Nations and the Agency for International Development, have selected and trained physicians, scientists, and many others in institutions that have created courses of study entirely for the benefit of other countries. Many of these programs have been highly successful; none has confused such carefully defined education with employment in the host country, delivery of services as a substitute for education, or permanent migration.

United States government-sponsored training for participants from developing countries has an excellent record of repatriation, as has that of the World Health Organization. Both are highly respected. The changes we have proposed certainly would not be attractive to hospitals that depend on FMGs to carry out essential hospital-based duties, but those hospitals should be prohibited from such practices, even without the proposed changes.

Foreign medical graduates who wish to become permanent residents and practice in the United States should be given the freedom to pursue their own interests. This choice should be restricted to those who possess Permanent Resident visas. Every effort should be made to evaluate their professional competence and to obtain proof that they meet the standards required of USMGs. As noted before, there is no substitute for graduation from medical schools that the United States medical profession regulates and approves. Continued acceptance of physicians who were graduated from foreign institutions throws a heavy burden on the testing mechanisms that are used as a substitute for the evaluations derived from the years of successful participation in our system of education. At present the National Board of Medical Examiners offers the most expert and acceptable series of examinations, although even these are based on the knowledge that the candidate was graduated from a medical school in the United States or Canada. Certainly nothing less than the full National Board examination should be used to determine the fitness of a physician to enter our health care system. If we demand it of our own graduates, there is no logic in not demanding it of those who are even less likely to be qualified to serve as house officers or to practice medicine independently.

Those states that have a keen interest in greater use of FMGs may, if they find this level of testing too harsh, set up supplementary educational programs to bring FMGs up to the level of their own graduates. This could be done through their medical schools at much less cost than for a full four years of education. Conceivably, the savings derived from these programs might be used to help educate the other FMGs who are going home again, or to support United States faculty participation in medical school teaching abroad.

Those FMGs who are here as Exchange Visitors could also enter the permanent resident system, but only by passing the same tests and by obtaining the graduate education required by the state.

Evaluation of permanent resident FMGs should not end at the point of entry into graduate medical education. There is no question about the limitations inherent in any examination system. One limitation is the fact that an examination measures knowledge only at a given point in time. Medical skills are cumulative, and the need for continued learning is well established. Every FMG who intends to remain here should serve an internship. Direct appointment to a residency should not be allowed. Thereafter, at each stage in his intended advancement to greater responsibility, his abilities should be carefully reevaluated to determine whether or not he has made adequate progress. If he has not done well enough he should be given further training at the level of his needs or dropped without having received a certificate of satisfactory performance.[5] Admittedly, this procedure will have meaning only when the FMG has not yet been licensed to practice, but the various state boards of medical examiners may take increasing cognizance of careful, professionally guided reports. Once the decision has been made to accept the physician as a potential member of our medical community, there should be no diminution of efforts to provide him with the assistance he needs to participate unrestrictedly in our health care system.

The recommendations are logical if our goals are those listed above. The FMG, the institutions he will serve, and the people of his country will benefit. The FMG who remains in the United States permanently will enter our health care system as a fully qualified physician, rather than at a second-class level, thereby assuring higher-quality health care for his patients.

Unquestionably, these changes would work a hardship on hospitals that are unwilling or unable to provide strong enough teaching programs to attract USMGs. This will exaggerate the inadequacies resulting from this country's manpower shortages, but we can find no justification in the current exploitative practices.

A further advantage to the medical profession will be the rededication of its organizations to the principles they have always supported. The inadvertent errors of the past two decades cannot be corrected painlessly. It will require great courage for the AMA, the AAMC, and the AHA to burden already beleaguered hospitals with a reduction in their supply of convenient and inexpensive help. It will require equal courage for them to maintain vigorous support of the policies and the regulatory mechanisms needed to assure successful results. The disruptive effects of these changes would be great primarily because we already import so many FMGs. Further delay will only aggravate the problems and increase the pressure on all medical institutions to make the adjustments that are already overdue. We are in trouble because we have drifted into indefensible and unsuccessful devices for meeting health needs that continue to grow. The issue should no longer be evaded.

COLLECTION AND DISSEMINATION OF DATA

The social phenomena summarized in this monograph have occurred almost unobserved. Regardless of any other improvements, the United States cannot again risk the mischances of obscurity. While the present abuses of laws and institutions were not predicted, there is no guarantee that new problems will not arise or that further modifications will not be needed. The INS should establish procedures that allow it to collect and publish data on FMGs, including their location in this country, their duration of stay, and their departures. This can be done more satisfactorily if the INS uses automated techniques, an obvious advantage in any modern system for data collection and analysis. Automation would also encourage the collection of additional information that is now unavailable from any source. This could include facts regarding employment in the country or origin, results of ECFMG examinations, commitments of FMGs to their own country, and duration of previous stay in the United States or a third country. The professional organizations that have accepted the responsibility for educating and evaluating FMGs should have INS reports fully available to them at all times.

THE RESPONSIBILITIES OF OTHER COUNTRIES

We have concentrated our attention on the policies and practices of this country. Obviously, the migration of physicians is

97

of concern to the governments of many countries, not excluding those that are relatively affluent. With few exceptions, record-keeping elsewhere has been less adequate than in the United Stats. The most common response to the problem of excessive migration of physicians has been the issuance of accusatory, propagandistic statements, usually devoid of facts. The United States can do nothing about India's or Pakistan's losses to England, but those countries can do much to counter their losses by more prudent planning at home. Except in a few countries like Colombia, realistic assessments of health manpower resources and needs in less developed countries are virtually nonexistent. These countries all recognize officially the high priority that should be given to preventive community health services, but their programing and budgeting are directed elsewhere. In general, medical education in the less developed countries emulates Western clinically oriented patterns, often with emphasis on the most expensive hospital procedures rather than on the massive infectious-disease problems with which they are burdened. Ministries of health are given a niggardly portion of the national budgets, which they too frequently invest in facilities that are available to only a small segment of the population. Salaries supplemented by income from private practice favor surgeons or physicians rather than public health officers, and those who serve rural communities have almost no opportunities for further training or other professional advancement. Medical schools may be created for political or prestige reasons without due regard for the capacity of the country or region to employ its graduates effectively.

Very little has been done to identify those physicians who might be interested in returning to their own countries from positions abroad. Only recently has the British government made any real effort to encourage repatriation of its physicians. Many FMGs do not even receive replies to their inquiries about positions available at home. Countries desperately in need of various kinds of specialists have no information about the qualifications and availability of their own citizens who are abroad. The World Health Organization, itself a beneficiary of physician migration, has contributed almost nothing to a better understanding of these issues although it is in an excellent position to do so.

LONG-TERM EVALUATION

Finally, there is a need for extensive studies of the fate of FMGs who have studied abroad and then returned to their own countries. The relevance of graduate education in this country to professional duties at home is still a matter of guesswork despite the years of effort that have gone into it. So long as our institutions attempt to serve the needs of other societies they must have some method for evaluating the results, using criteria other than those we use for our own society. This can be done by follow-up observations conducted by the AAMC or another professional organization that is competent to evaluate both medical education and its application in a variety of health care systems.

APPENDIX A   Supplement to Chapter II

A BRIEF HISTORY OF THE ECFMG

Prior to the Second World War, few foreign nationals came to this country for advanced medical training, and many United States citizens pursued their advanced training in European schools. After the war, however, United States hospitals entered a period of rapid growth. They expanded their internship and residency programs until in 1958 there were nearly twice as many positions available as there were USMGs to fill them. At the same time salaries for house staff members began rising. Concomitantly, in 1948 the United States government began its cultural exchange program, and Fulbright funds for travel soon became available for foreign physicians who wished to train in this country. American medicine and technological advances were beginning to outpace the rest of the world by a considerable margin. Entry into the United States was becoming easier, if not on a permanent basis, at least with an Exchange visa which in the 1950's was valid for one year but could be renewed year after year. The result was a favorable combination of circumstances for FMGs. By the early 1950's it became apparent that hospitals were obtaining FMGs whose credentials they often could not understand, let alone validate, whose command of English was poor, and whose knowledge of medicine was often inadequate. Many hospitals neglected to give FMGs the proper orientation, burdened them with too many menial tasks, and expected more than the FMGs could produce. The situation became alarming. Consequently, in 1954 responsible officials from the AHA, the AMA, the Federation of State Medical Boards, and the AAMC met and established a "Cooperating

103

Committee on Graduates of Foreign Medical Schools." [1] Three representatives from each of the aforementioned groups were members of this Committee, which was set up to study the problems of FMGs and to make recommendations for their resolution.

In the years between 1954 and 1957, the Cooperating Committee met many times and eventually evolved a plan which called for the establishment of an Educational Council for Foreign Medical Graduates (ECFMG). The proposed ECFMG would be an independent organization governed by a ten-man Board of Trustees composed of two representatives each from the AHA, AMA, AAMC, and the Federation of State Medical Examiners, plus two members from the public at large.

The founders of the ECFMG originally envisioned its duties as including three specific functions and two general ones. The specific functions were information, evaluation, and certification. The ECFMG's general functions were "to give graduates of foreign medical schools an opportunity to establish, while still in their own country, their qualifications for undertaking advanced medical training as interns or residents in U.S. hospitals," and "to provide hospitals, State Boards of Medical Examiners, and Specialty Boards with a means of identifying (a) those FMGs who can safely be considered on the same basis as graduates of United States medical schools, (b) those FMGs who, though not fully equivalent to United States students, are qualified to assume, for a period not to exceed two years, places as interns and *assistant* residents in United States hospitals; and (c) those FMGs who are not yet ready to assume internship or *assistant* residency positions in U.S. hospitals." [2]

While the Cooperating Committee was still formulating its policy prior to establishing the ECFMG, it estimated the number of candidates who were likely to apply annually to take the ECFMG examination. The Committee assumed that there would be approximately 500 applicants in the United States each year, 400 of whom would be eligible to take the examination; and that there would be approximately 3000 applicants from abroad, 1000 of whom would be successful in passing the examination

104

and receiving a hospital appointment in this country.[3] On the basis of these estimates, arrangements were made to begin the operations of the ECFMG in 1957. A schedule of fees was worked out, and a small staff began to implement the policy decisions of the Cooperating Committee.

In its report of May 10, 1956, the Cooperating Committee also established the criteria for evaluating medical credentials. The "basic requirements" were:

1. A minimum of 18 years of formal education.
2. Included in this minimum of 18 years of formal education should be a minimum of 32 months of attendance at a school of medicine, and direct study of medicine, excluding any time devoted to what in the United States would be considered as premedical study or internship.
3. In any country where the minimum standards stated above do not constitute sufficient educational achievement to acquire licensure in that country, the latter rather than the minimum previously described would be required. Although it would be expected that licensure would be achieved in the country in which is located the school of graduation, under exceptional circumstances such licensure would not be demanded if the candidate had fulfilled all of the educational requirements for licensure.
4. Evidence of satisfactory completion of the above-described courses of study.
5. As evidence of acceptable moral and ethical behavior, each candidate must present a properly executed affidavit that he has not been convicted of any crime involving moral turpitude and that he has never been censured or had any other punitive action taken against him for reasons of immoral conduct by a recognized medical body, including licensing agencies.

Two exceptions were made to the above-listed requirements. One involved the allowance of secondary evidence for displaced persons who were not able to produce their original credentials, and the other allowed foreign-trained physicians who are considered to be properly qualified for the practice of medicine by a state licensing board to be admitted to an approved internship or residency program.[4]

Under the plan established by the Cooperating Committee, an ECFMG Examination Committee was set up which was entrusted with the responsibility of making up the ECFMG examination from a pool of questions from the National Board of Medical Examiners. The Educational Testing Service of Princeton was originally chosen to arrange the administration of the ECFMG examination, but the National Board of Medical Examiners insisted upon direct control of the ECFMG examining procedures if its pool of questions was to be used. The Board of Trustees subsequently agreed to this arrangement. Therefore, the National Board of Medical Examiners was given the authority to set up the examination centers and to proctor, score, and tabulate the examinations.

THE FIRST ECFMG EXAMINATIONS

On March 25, 1958, the first ECFMG examination was administered in seventeen United States and Canadian medical schools. At that time, 298 FMGs took the examination, and 151 of them (51 percent) passed it. The first examination, consisting of 400 multiple-choice questions, was given in two three-hour sessions on the same day, with one-half hour at the beginning of the afternoon sessions devoted to an English test. Originally, this ECFMG examination was called the "American Medical Qualification Examination," since the questions on it were derived from the pool of questions provided by the National Board of Medical Examiners. The English portion of the original examination was designed to test the candidate's writing ability and understanding of spoken English. It was assumed that, if a candidate could pass the written examination, this was sufficient evidence of his ability to read and understand written English. Consequently, the English examination *per se* consisted of listening to a patient state his medical history, then listening to the proctor read this same medical history, taking notes, and summarizing the history in a ten-minute résumé.

Since there were 151 FMGs who scored 75 percent or higher

106

on the first examination, the results were considered disappointing. This was primarily because all of those (298) who took the test had had between 1 and 20 years of previous experience with medicine in the United States, and the questions selected were ones that would be the least likely to confuse an FMG.

Between the first and second ECFMG examinations, several important decisions were made and events occurred. In the summer of 1958, the ECFMG established 27 examination centers overseas. It also made a policy decision not to lower the passing score to 70 percent because the ECFMG could then no longer "state that the certified physicians had reached a level of educational attainment comparable with that of a graduate of the United States schools." At the same time, a decision was made to issue "temporary certificates" to those FMGs who scored between 70 and 74 percent with a provision that they must retake and pass the ECFMG examination if they planned to remain in a United States training program for longer than two years.

Shortly after the results of the first ECFMG examination were known, many hospital administrators began to express concern that its introduction would seriously diminish the flow of foreign physicians to this country. At the AHA's annual convention in August 1958 it was suggested that "the AHA take steps to defer, if at all possible," the inclusion of FMGs in the intern matching program and "examine and test the present mechanism in view of the high percentage of failures." [5]

On another front, complaints were beginning to be heard from FMGs who had taken the examination. They were unhappy over the length of the examination, the complexity of the system of multiple-choice questions, and the high score necessary for passing. With the exception of the decision to issue temporary certificates, however, no major changes were made prior to the second examination, which was given on September 23, 1958 in 30 centers in the United States and 27 others throughout the world.

The number of FMGs who wrote the second examination was almost three times the number who took the first one, but the passing rate remained almost the same. Since temporary certificates were issued, the ECFMG estimated that between 50 and 60 percent of the FMGs who took the American Qualification Examination would continue to qualify for internships and residencies in United States hospitals.

By 1959, the number of FMGs who were qualified and certified by the ECFMG had quadrupled. Then, in 1960, a period of phenomenal growth began. That year a total of 14,768 FMGs wrote the examination, and since 1963 it has been taken by an average of 18,700 FMGs annually. Since the budget for 1959 had been based upon an estimated 5200 applicants, the number of candidates from 1960 on was vastly different from what had been anticipated. Tables A1 and A2 show in detail the experience of the ECFMG examination over a nine-year period.

SUBSEQUENT REVISIONS OF THE ECFMG

There have been several modifications in the structure of the ECFMG over the course of the past several years, involving the changes outlined below.

The Examination. In 1959 the number of questions on the ECFMG examination was reduced from 400 to 360, and in 1962 the use of the name "American Medical Qualification Examination" was discontinued. The new name became "the ECFMG Examination."

The English portion of the ECFMG examination proved to be unsatisfactory and in October 1963 a new system of testing was instituted. Under the old system, a candidate was required to write a short case history in English after he had listened to a proctor read a patient's history. The English examination that has been given since October 1963 consists of a 50-item multiple-choice examination in which the candidate listens to a proctor as he reads certain words or short narratives and then selects the correct answers from a series of alternatives.

Educational Requirements. As a result of its experiences with the extreme variations among the countries of the world in their medical education requirements, the Board of Trustees of the ECFMG voted in 1964 to modify its educational requirements.

Table A1. ECFMG Examination, March, 1958-September, 1966. Summary of results

	Mar. 25 1958	Sept. 23 1958	Feb. 19 1959	Sept. 22 1959	Mar. 16 1960	Sept. 21 1960	Apr. 4 1961	Oct. 17 1961	Mar. 28 1962	Oct. 24 1962
Number Taking Examination, by Domestic and Foreign Examination Centers										
Examination Centers										
Domestic	298	707	1,278	2,351	4,909	7,308	5,326	3,204	3,034	2,879
Foreign	—	137	494	717	1,146	1,405	2,500	3,192	3,320	5,302
Total	298	844	1,772	3,068	6,055	8,713	7,826	6,396	6,354	8,181
% Foreign	(0.0)	(16.2)	(27.9)	(23.4)	(18.9)	(16.1)	(31.9)	(49.9)	(52.3)	(64.8)
Scoring 75 or Higher										
Dom. - No.	152	371	616	1,088	1,650	3,222	2,063	1,079	1,164	1,154
%	(51.0)	(52.4)	(48.2)	(46.3)	(33.6)	(44.1)	(38.7)	(33.7)	(38.4)	(40.1)
For. - No.	—	47	153	282	347	554	1,040	1,199	1,625	2,111
%	(—)	(31.0)	(31.0)	(39.3)	(30.3)	(39.4)	(46.6)	(37.6)	(48.9)	(39.8)
Tot. - No.	152	418	769	1,370	1,997	3,776	3,103	2,278	2,789	3,265
%	(51.0)	(49.5)	(43.4)	(44.7)	(33.0)	(43.3)	(39.6)	(35.6)	(43.9)	(39.9)
Number Taking Examination, by Number of Times Tested										
Number of Times Tested										
First Exam	298	796	1,644	2,833	5,278	6,023	4,501	3,703	3,483	5,423
Repeat Exam	—	48	128	235	777	2,690	3,325	2,693	2,871	2,758
Total	298	844	1,772	3,068	6,055	8,713	7,826	6,396	6,354	8,181
% Taking First Exam	(100)	(94.3)	(92.8)	(92.3)	(87.2)	(69.1)	(57.5)	(57.9)	(54.8)	(66.3)

109

Table A1 - continued

	Mar. 27 1963	Oct. 23 1963	Mar. 25 1964	Oct. 21 1964	Mar. 24 1965	Sept. 15 1965	Feb. 9 1966	Sept. 14 1966	Totals
	Number Taking Examination, by Domestic and Foreign Examination Centers - continued								
Examination Centers									
Domestic	2,911	3,143	2,813	2,899	2,995	2,083	2,006	1,919	52,063
Foreign	5,461	7,615	6,032	6,767	6,853	6,406	7,020	8,043	72,410
Total	8,372	10,758	8,845	9,666	9,848	8,489	9,026	9,962	124,473
% Foreign	(65.2)	(70.8)	(68.2)	(70.0)	(69.6)	(75.5)	(77.8)	(80.7)	(58.2)
	Scoring 75 or Higher - continued								
Dom. - No.	884	1,016	1,120	996	1,373	888	722	655	20,213
%	(30.4)	(32.3)	(39.8)	(34.4)	(45.8)	(42.6)	(36.0)	(34.1)	(38.8)
For. - No.	1,859	2,284	2,505	2,199	2,797	2,666	2,790	3,675	28,133
%	(34.0)	(30.0)	(41.5)	(32.5)	(40.8)	(41.6)	(39.7)	(45.7)	(38.9)
Tot. - No.	2,743	3,300	3,625	3,195	4,170	3,554	3,512	4,330	48,346
%	(32.8)	(30.7)	(41.0)	(33.1)	(42.3)	(41.9)	(38.9)	(43.5)	(38.8)
	Number Taking Examination, by Number of Times Tested - continued								
Number of Times Tested									
First Exam	5,032	6,359	4,559	4,819	4,799	4,405	4,864	5,901	74,720
Repeat Exam	3,340	4,399	4,286	4,847	5,049	4,084	4,162	4,061	49,753
Total	8,372	10,758	8,845	9,666	9,848	8,489	9,026	9,962	124,473
% Taking First Exam	(60.1)	(59.1)	(51.5)	(49.9)	(48.7)	(51.9)	(53.9)	(59.2)	(60.0)

Source: Reproduced from ECFMG *Annual Report*, 1966, p. 9. Used by permission of the ECFMG.

Table A2. ECFMG Examinations, March, 1958-September, 1966. Summary of results obtained by individual candidates

	March 25 1958	Sept. 23 1958	Feb. 19 1959	Sept. 22 1959	Mar. 16 1960	Sept. 21 1960	Apr. 4 1961	Oct. 17 1961
1. Total number	298	844	1,772	3,068	6,055	8,713	7,826	6,396
2. First-timers	298	796	1,644	2,833	5,278	6,023	4,501	3,703
3. Cumulative First-timers	298	1,094	2,738	5,571	10,849	16,872	21,373	25,076
4. Number scoring 75 or higher	152	418	769	1,370	1,997	3,776	3,103	2,278
5. Per cent scoring 75 or higher	51.0	49.5	43.4	44.7	33.0	43.3	39.6	35.6
6. Cumulative total 75 or higher	152	570	1,339	2,709	4,706	8,482	11,585	13,836
7. Cumulative per cent scoring 75 or higher	51.0	52.1	48.9	48.6	43.4	50.3	54.2	55.2

Table A2 - continued

	Mar. 28 1962	Oct. 27 1962	Mar. 27 1963	Oct. 23 1963	March 25 1964	Oct. 21 1964	March 24 1965	Sept. 15 1965	Feb. 9 1966	Sept. 14 1966
1. Total number	6,354	8,181	8,372	10,758	8,845	9,666	9,848	8,489	9,026	9,962
2. First-timers	3,483	5,423	5,032	6,359	4,559	4,819	4,799	4,405	4,864	5,901
3. Cumulative First-timers	28,559	33,982	39,014	45,373	49,932	54,751	59,550	63,955	68,619	74,720
4. Number scoring 75 or higher	2,789	3,265	2,743	3,300	3,625	3,195	4,170	3,554	3,512	4,330
5. Per cent scoring 75 or higher	43.9	39.9	32.8	30.7	41.0	33.1	42.3	41.9	38.9	43.5
6. Cumulative total 75 or higher	16,652	19,917	22,660	25,960	29,585	32,780	36,950	40,504	44,016	48,346
7. Cumulative per cent scoring 75 or higher	58.3	58.6	58.1	57.2	59.2	59.9	62.0	63.3	64.0	64.7

Source: ECFMG *Annual Report*, 1966, p. 9. Used by permission of the ECFMG.

APPENDIX A

It abolished the requirement that a candidate for ECFMG certification have at least 18 years of formal education and substituted the stipulation that an FMG have a full and unrestricted license to practice medicine in his own country. The Board additionally voted not to apply this licensure requirement to graduates of Italian medical schools who would receive the *Laurea in Medicina e Chirugia* prior to July 1, 1966, or to graduates of Commonwealth and United Kingdom schools, or of German and Mexican schools under various conditions.

Policy on Temporary Certificates. Under considerable pressure, the Board of Trustees voted in 1958 to issue Temporary Certificates to those FMGs who came within five points of obtaining the passing score of 75 percent on the ECFMG Examination. By 1962, it became apparent that the disadvantages of such a policy were great, and a longitudinal study of candidates with Temporary Certificates was begun in 1963. As a result of this study, it was found that the benefits derived from certification on a temporary basis were not sufficient to warrant the continuation of the policy. Therefore, at the end of 1963 the Board of Trustees voted to stop the issuance of Temporary Certificates after the examination of March 25, 1964, and the last of these certificates expired on June 30, 1966.

On December 8 and 9, 1960, a Conference on International Education in Medicine convened in Washington. Out of that conference, and from the Steering Committee which the Conference appointed, came several recommendations that were submitted as proposals to the Board of Trustees of the ECFMG. These proposals had been debated and formulated by an outstanding group representing the AMA, AAMC, AHA, PHS, Rockefeller Foundation, and the State Department, who were genuinely concerned with the mounting problems in United States medical education.

The Steering Committee made eight recommendations for the strengthening of the ECFMG. They included the development of: (1) better informational facilities; (2) orientation services; (3) better selection methods; (4) special preparatory training services; (5) consultation services with hospitals and counseling

113

for FMGs; (6) special residency programs for selected FMGs in the United States and USMGs abroad; (7) liaison with governmental and nongovernmental agencies for their active participation; (8) a special appraisal service to study the utilization of FMGs and the effectiveness of their training in United States hospitals.

In 1962, the Board of Trustees voted to accept the following six-point statement of the main purposes of the ECFMG:

1. To promote the advanced study of medicine in the United States of America by graduates of foreign medical schools and thereby to assist those graduates in raising the level of medical care and medical education of other countries.

2. To expand, for graduates of foreign medical schools, the educational opportunity in hospitals in the United States.

3. To serve the public interest by a program of education, testing, and evaluation of foreign-trained physicians which will help assure the public that such physicians are properly qualified to assume responsibility for the care of patients as interns or residents in hospitals in the United States.

4. To evaluate the educational qualifications and medical training of foreign physicians who desire to further their education in the United States and with respect thereto, to verify credentials, to arrange, supervise and conduct examinations to determine the readiness of such individuals to benefit from education as interns or residents in United States hospitals.

5. To disseminate information and data among graduates of foreign medical schools relating to the problems, requirements and procedures for residents and interns in hospitals in the United States and thereby enable them to prepare to obtain maximum benefit from these hospital programs.

6. To assist in the continued improvement of the medical educational programs and standards of hospitals in the United States.[6]

In its Philadelphia offices, the ECFMG today is staffed with more than thirty full-time employees. The original founding members — the AMA, AHA, and AAMC, the Federation of State Boards of Medical Examiners, and the public at large — constitute the Board of Trustees. An IBM computer processed over 22,000 applications for ECFMG examinations in 1966, and there are over 98,000 applications on which the Council maintains active files. Recently, in Manila, the ECFMG examination was given in a football stadium to accommodate the huge number of applicants. There are no indications that the volume of applicants is decreasing.

APPENDIX B Selected Data on FMGs

in the United States

116

117

APPENDIX B

TABLE B1. Physicians and surgeons admitted as Permanent Residents, fiscal years 1957-1964

Country	1957	1958	1959	1960	1961	1962	1963	1964
Europe	871	781	726	550	553	502	575	623
Austria	67	24	27	16	11	6	15	14
Belgium	9	10	9	8	17	12	16	15
Bulgaria	0	0	1	0	0	0	1	1
Czechoslovakia	1	1	1	0	1	0	1	0
Denmark	6	0	5	3	2	5	4	4
Estonia	0	0	0	0	0	1	0	0
Finland	2	0	1	0	0	2	2	1
France	32	32	32	25	14	25	24	34
Germany	206	128	95	75	77	73	71	82
Greece	61	53	23	37	32	31	31	30
Hungary	40	34	136	37	27	2	0	2
Iceland	0	0	0	0	2	3	1	2
Ireland	48	54	47	56	22	21	27	23
Italy	119	82	66	49	39	47	49	22
Latvia	0	1	0	0	2	0	0	0
Luxembourg	3	0	0	1	0	0	0	2
Malta	1	1	0	0	0	0	0	0
Netherlands	41	32	29	31	28	14	16	15
Norway	3	0	5	5	1	1	1	3
Poland	2	7	12	20	23	16	10	19
Portugal	5	6	0	1	3	3	1	4
Rumania	0	0	0	1	1	3	1	4
Spain	23	32	22	17	23	47	47	108
Sweden	6	8	11	5	9	10	9	7
Switzerland	33	32	27	21	29	21	28	31
Turkey	17	48	19	10	43	31	55	29
U.S.S.R.	1	1	2	2	1	0	1	1
Yugoslavia	3	6	9	5	6	9	10	5
United Kingdom	142	189	147	125	140	119	154	165
England	113	158	118	96	116	98	133	137
No. Ireland	9	13	14	6	9	6	3	6
Scotland	18	16	12	18	15	13	15	18
Wales	2	2	3	5	0	2	3	4
Canada	256	218	210	245	287	280	467	440
Mexico	95	57	44	66	64	70	97	77
British West Indies	4	6	8	10	7	–	–	–
Cuba	199	86	77	94	94	120	156	229
South America	228	285	227	256	208	298	327	454
Asia	155	316	207	244	269	265	260	204
All other	182	185	131	109	201	262	211	222
Total	1990	1934	1630	1574	1683	1797	2093	2249

Source: United States Department of Justice, Immigration and Naturalization Service

TABLE B2. Numbers of physicians and surgeons admitted as Exchange Visitors, fiscal year 1966.

Country or region of last residence	Physicians and surgeons
Developed countries	<u>1,743</u>
Europe	<u>881</u>
Austria	15
Belgium	32
Denmark	20
Finland	19
France	41
Germany	155
Greece	31
Ireland	20
Italy	80
Netherlands	23
Norway	15
Portugal	10
Spain	61
Sweden	64
Switzerland	58
United Kingdom	174
Other Europe	103
Asia	<u>423</u>
Japan	423
North America	<u>339</u>
Canada	339
Africa	<u>32</u>
South Africa	32
Oceania	<u>68</u>
Australia	51
New Zealand	17

TABLE B2 - continued

Country or region of last residence	Physicians and surgeons
Developing countries	2,627
Europe	15
Turkey (includes Asia)	15
Asia	2,120
Burma	3
China (includes Taiwan)	92
Hong Kong	36
India	444
Indonesia	5
Iran	105
Iraq	24
Israel	68
Jordan (includes Arab Palestine)	10
Korea	291
Lebanon	28
Malaysia	14
Pakistan	69
Philippines	754
Syrian Arab Republic	19
Thailand	128
Vietnam	12
Other Asia	18
North America	207
Mexico	131
Other North America	2
Dominican Republic	5
Haiti	3
Other West Indies	28
Costa Rica	8
El Salvador	7
Guatemala	10

TABLE B2 - continued

Country or region of last residence	Physicians and surgeons
North America (Cont'd)	
Honduras	4
Nicaragua	2
Panama	6
Other Central America	1
South America	211
Argentina	58
Bolivia	1
Brazil	40
Chile	12
Colombia	35
Ecuador	1
Paraguay	10
Peru	15
Uruguay	6
Venezuela	29
Other South America	4
Africa	66
Algeria	1
Ethiopia	2
Ghana	5
Kenya	4
Morocco	—
Nigeria	9
Tunisia	1
U.A.R. (Egypt)	24
Other Africa	20
All Other Countries	8
Total, all countries	4,370

Source: United States Department of Justice, Immigration and Naturalization Service, April 4, 1967.

Table B3 . Immigration of scientists, engineers, and medical personnel, fiscal year 1966

Country or region of last residence	Total	Medical Personnel			
		Physicians and surgeons	Dentists	Nurses	
				Professional	Student
All countries	6,335	2,552	209	3,430	144
Developed countries	3,722	1,075	72	2,459	116
Europe	1,932	613	54	1,209	56
Austria	49	16	5	28	0
Belgium	34	17	2	15	0
Denmark	41	2	1	33	5
Finland	13	3	0	10	0
France	61	24	3	30	4
Germany	252	81	5	156	10
Greece	53	38	2	12	1
Ireland	134	22	2	108	2
Italy	70	43	4	23	0
Netherlands	55	11	0	44	0
Norway	73	6	4	60	3
Portugal	10	4	0	4	2
Spain	81	56	10	13	2
Sweden	94	20	2	63	9
Switzerland	63	27	1	35	0
United Kingdom	732	187	5	523	17
Other Europe	117	56	8	52	1
Asia	45	31	1	13	0
Japan	45	31	1	13	0

Table B3 - continued

Country or region of last residence	Total	Medical Personnel		Nurses	
		Physicians and surgeons	Dentists	Professional	Student
Asia (Continued)					
Korea	54	35	0	17	2
Lebanon	25	14	2	9	0
Malaysia	10	5	0	5	0
Pakistan	11	11	0	0	0
Philippines	419	259	21	137	2
Syrian Arab Republic	11	9	0	2	0
Thailand	47	11	0	35	1
Vietnam	7	1	0	6	0
Other Asia	8	5	0	3	0
North America	993	462	58	457	16
Mexico	170	119	9	41	1
Other North America	65	49	4	9	3
Dominican Republic	91	59	6	26	0
Haiti	62	29	6	26	1
Other West Indies	471	177	30	257	7
Costa Rica	17	3	1	13	0
El Salvador	22	4	0	16	2
Guatemala	31	8	0	22	1
Honduras	25	4	1	19	1
Nicaragua	13	6	0	7	0
Panama	12	3	0	9	0
Other Central Amer.	14	1	1	12	0

123

Table B3 - continued

Country or region of last residence	Total	Medical Personnel			Nurses	
		Physicians and surgeons	Dentists		Professional	Student
North America	1,660	393	16		1,193	58
Canada	1,660	393	16		1,193	58
Africa	22	15	1		6	0
South Africa	22	15	1		6	0
Oceania	63	23	0		38	2
Australia	54	21	0		32	1
New Zealand	9	2	0		6	1
Developing countries	2,613	1,477	137		971	28
Europe	61	57	0		4	0
Turkey (includes Asia)	61	57	0		4	0
Asia	913	557	32		314	10
Burma	7	5	0		2	0
China (includes Taiwan)	35	16	1		18	0
Hong Kong	71	26	3		38	4
India	50	40	2		7	1
Indonesia	0	0	0		0	0
Iran	86	78	2		6	0
Iraq	7	5	0		2	0
Israel	58	31	1		26	0
Jordan (includes Arab Palestine)	7	6	0		1	0

Table B3 - continued

Country or region of last residence	Total	Medical Personnel		Nurses	
		Physicians and surgeons	Dentists	Professional	Student
South America	576	355	44	175	2
Argentina	151	115	11	25	0
Bolivia	24	19	3	2	0
Brazil	57	33	9	15	0
Chile	24	11	1	12	0
Colombia	123	80	10	33	0
Ecuador	57	23	4	29	1
Paraguay	6	6	0	0	0
Peru	64	46	1	17	0
Uruguay	12	7	2	3	0
Venezuela	19	11	3	5	0
Other South America	39	4	0	34	1
Africa	67	45	3	19	0
Algeria	3	2	0	1	0
Ethiopia	4	4	0	0	0
Ghana	2	0	0	2	0
Kenya	2	1	0	1	0
Morocco	5	2	0	3	0
Nigeria	3	2	0	1	0
Tunisia	2	2	0	0	0
U.A.R. (Egypt)	27	23	2	2	0
Other Africa	19	9	1	9	0
All other countries	3	1	0	2	0

Source: United States Department of Justice, Immigration and Naturalization Service, April 4, 1967.

Table B4. Status of internship and residency programs in the United States, 1941-1967

Year	Total offered	Total filled	Internships					Total vacant
			Filled by non-foreign graduates	Filled by foreign graduates	Filled federal services[a]			
					V.A.	Other		
1966-67	13,569	10,366	7,573	2,793	73	663		3,203
1965-66	12,954	9,670	7,309	2,361	93	613		3,284
1964-65	12,728	10,097	7,276	2,821	46	563		2,631
1963-64	12,229	9,636	7,070	2,566	45	569		2,593
1962-63	12,024	8,805	7,136	1,669	41	533		3,219
1961-62	12,074	8,173	6,900	1,273	42	581		3,901
1960-61	12,547	9,115	7,362	1,753	71	576		3,432
1959-60	12,580	10,253	7,708	2,545	55	584		2,327
1958-59	12,469	10,352	8,037	2,315	25	567		2,117
1957-58	12,325	10,198	8,119	2,079	48	566		2,127
1956-57	11,895	9,893	7,905	1,988	58	532		2,002
1955-56	11,616	9,603	7,744	1,859	55	495		2,013
1954-55	11,048	9,066	7,305	1,761	88	470		1,982
1953-54	10,542	8,275	6,488	1,787	88	433		2,267
1952-53	10,548	7,645	6,292	1,353	67	393		2,903
1951-52	10,044	7,866	6,750	1,116	71	472		2,178
1950-51	9,370	7,030	6,308	722	—	435		2,340
1949-50	9,124	7,313	—	b	—	—		1,811
1948-49	9,027	7,248	—	—	—	—		1,779
1947-48	8,683	6,902	—	—	—	—		1,781
1946-47	8,584	—	—	—	—	—		—
1945-46	8,429	—	—	—	—	—		—
World War II 1941-1942	8,182	—	—	—	—	—		—

Table B4 - continued

Residencies

Year	Total offered	Total filled	Filled by non-foreign graduates	Filled by foreign graduates	Filled federal services[a]		Total vacant
					V.A.	Other	
1966-67	39,384	32,050	22,548	9,502	1,590	1,548	7,334
1965-66	38,979	31,898	22,765	9,133	1,753	1,352	7,074
1964-65	38,750	31,005	22,852	8,153	2,127	1,353	7,749
1963-64	37,357	29,485	22,433	7,052	2,104	1,338	7,728
1962-63	36,502	29,239	22,177	7,062	2,464	1,223	7,263
1961-62	35,403	29,637	21,914	7,723	2,602	1,249	5,766
1960-61	32,786	28,447	20,265	8,182	2,830	1,177	4,339
1959-60	31,733	27,590	20,619	6,912	2,650	1,456	4,143
1958-59	31,818	26,758	20,716	6,042	2,453	1,267	5,060
1957-58	30,595	24,976	19,433	5,543	2,403	1,049	5,619
1956-57	28,528	23,012	18,259	4,753	2,304	1,276	5,516
1955-56	26,516	21,425	17,251	4,174	2,353	624	5,091
1954-55	25,486	20,494	17,219	3,275	2,252	657	4,992
1953-54	23,630	18,619	14,817	3,802	2,072	639	5,011
1952-53	22,292	16,867	13,832	3,035	2,021	768	5,425
1951-52	20,645	15,851	13,618	2,233	2,120	761	4,794
1950-51	19,364	14,495	13,145	1,350	—	—	4,869
1949-50	18,669	17,490	—	b	—	—	1,179
1948-49	17,293	—	—	—	—	—	—
1947-48	15,172	—	—	—	—	—	—
1946-47	12,003	—	—	—	c	—	—
1945-46	8,930	—	—	—	—	—	—
World War II							
1941-1942	5,256	—	—	—	—	—	—

Source: *JAMA, 202* (1967), 781. Used by permission of the *Journal of the American Medical Association.*

[a]Figures for filled Federal Services also included in three preceding columns.
[b]U.S. Information and Educational Exchange Act of 1946, effective July 1949.
[c]P. L. 293—Jan. 3, 1946—Authorizing Residency Programs in Veterans Administration.

TABLE B5. Range of salaries for interns and residents, 1968-1969

a. Annual internship salaries

Annual salary offered	Affiliated hospitals	Nonaffiliated hospitals	Total
Data Not Available	74	65	139
Not Applicable	1	0	1
0- 500	0	0	0
501- 1,000	0	0	0
1,001- 1,500	0	0	0
1,501- 2,000	3	0	3
2,001- 2,500	1	0	1
2,501- 3,000	64	9	73
3,001- 3,500	63	5	68
3,501- 4,000	342	244	586
4,001- 4,500	297	206	503
4,501- 5,000	122	249	371
5,001- 5,500	120	145	265
5,501- 6,000	132	137	269
6,001- 6,500	4	18	22
6,501- 7,000	0	32	32
7,001- 7,500	14	20	34
7,501- 8,000	1	1	2
8,001- 8,500	4	5	9
8,501- 9,000	0	0	0
9,001- 9,500	0	0	0
9,501-10,000	0	0	0
Over 10,000	0	0	0
Totals	**1,242**	**1,136**	**2,378**
Mean	$4,139	$4,521	$4,322
Median	$4,001-4,500	$5,001-5,500	$4,001-4,500
Mode	$3,501-4,000	$4,501-5,000	$3,501-4,000

Source: *JAMA, 202* (1967), 768. Used by permission of the *Journal of the American Medical Association.*

TABLE B5 - continued

b. Annual residency salaries

Annual salary offered	Affiliated hospitals	Nonaffiliated hospitals	Total
Data Not Available	229	230	459
0- 500	0	0	0
501- 1,000	0	0	0
1,001- 1,500	2	1	3
1,501- 2,000	1	1	2
2,001- 2,500	7	1	8
2,501- 3,000	31	3	34
3,001- 3,500	54	3	57
3,501- 4,000	306	121	427
4,001- 4,500	731	245	976
4,501- 5,000	957	384	1,341
5,001- 5,500	428	382	810
5,501- 6,000	285	291	576
6,001- 6,500	161	143	304
6,501- 7,000	115	116	231
7,001- 7,500	86	55	141
7,501- 8,000	32	44	76
8,001- 8,500	29	48	77
8,501- 9,000	13	37	50
9,001- 9,500	12	6	18
9,501-10,000	6	8	14
10,001-10,500	5	13	18
10,501-11,000	5	7	12
11,001-11,500	0	2	2
11,501-12,000	2	3	5
12,001-12,500	0	0	0
12,501-13,000	0	0	0
Over 13,000	2	2	4
Total	3,499	2,146	5,645
Mean	$4,095	$4,557	$4,295
Median	$4,501-5,000	$5,001-5,500	$4,501-5,000
Mode	$4,501-5,000	$4,501-5,000	$4,501-5,000

Source: *JAMA, 202* November (1967), 775. Used by permission of the *Journal of the American Medical Association.*

Table B6. Trends in annual salaries (dollars) for interns and residents, 1962-1968

	Interns		Residents	
Year	Average salaries	Change	Average salaries	Change
1 962-63	2,796		3,300	
1963-64	3,039	+243	3,684	+384
1964-65	3,425	+386	4,037	+353
1965-66	3,529	+104	3,989	- 48
1966-67	3,797	+268	3,931	- 58
1967-68	4,322	+529	4,295	+264

Source: *JAMA, 202* (1967), 775. Used by permission of the *Journal of the American Medical Association.*

Table B7. Foreign countries with medical schools contributing
the most graduates to U.S. graduate medical programs, December 31,
1966

Country	Total number of trainees	Percent of total foreign graduates in U.S. graduate programs
Philippines	3,517	26
India	1,468	11
Korea	805	6
Iran	612	4
Thailand	531	4
Cuba	462	3
Argentina	446	3
Mexico	385	3
Spain	371	3
Germany	360	3
Colombia	347	3
Italy	345	3
Taiwan	329	2
Switzerland	297	2
Total	**10,275**	**75**

Source: *JAMA, 202* (1967), 786. Used by permission of the *Journal of the American Medical Association.*

Table B8. Visa status of FMGs in U. S. graduate programs, December 31, 1966

Visa	Categories		
	Training	Research	Total
None	1,518	492	2,010
Permanent Resident	2,791	340	3,131
First Preference	15	7	22
Student	145	9	154
Exchange Visitor	8,783	276	9,059
Refugee or displaced person	109	2	111
Miscellaneous	46	11	57
Total	14,735	1,137	15,872

Source: *JAMA, 202* (1967), 786. Used by permission of the *Journal of the American Medical Association.*

Table B9. Distribution of foreign graduate trainees by country of medical education, December 31, 1966

Country of medical training	Interns	Residents	Total
Afghanistan	–	2	2
Argentina	74	372	446
Australia	6	69	75
Austria	12	55	67
Belgium	17	108	125
Bolivia	11	33	44
Brazil	19	73	92
Bulgaria	1	6	7
Burma	7	13	20
Ceylon	–	6	6
Chile	3	33	36
China	10	39	49
Colombia	38	309	347
Cuba	82	380	462
Czechoslovakia	11	28	39
Denmark	8	7	15
Dominican Republic	8	116	124
Ecuador	6	13	19
Egypt	20	97	117
El Salvador	5	12	17
England	15	146	161
Estonia	–	1	1
Finland	–	3	3
Formosa	69	260	329
France	8	64	72
Germany	75	285	360
Greece	15	105	120
Guatemala	11	57	68
Haiti	26	60	86
Honduras	1	7	8
Hong Kong	4	18	22
Hungary	3	27	30
Iceland	4	33	37
India	239	1,229	1,468
Indonesia	3	3	6
Iran	101	511	612
Iraq	21	62	83
Ireland	43	155	198
Israel	7	68	75
Italy	59	286	345
Japan	17	153	170
Korea	291	514	805
Latvia	–	4	4
Lebanon	12	114	126
Lithuania	–	1	1
Manchuria	–	3	3
Mexico	64	321	385

Table B9 - continued

Country of medical training	Interns	Residents	Total
The Netherlands	8	70	78
New Zealand	2	21	23
Nicaragua	1	11	12
Nigeria	3	3	6
Norway	–	2	2
Pakistan	50	238	288
Panama	2	14	16
Paraguay	4	16	20
Peru	41	112	153
Philipines	721	2,796	3,517
Poland	13	64	77
Portugal	2	29	31
Romania	17	74	91
Scotland	20	53	73
Singapore-Malaya	1	4	5
South Africa, Union of	3	83	86
South Vietnam	–	4	4
Spain	61	310	371
Surinam	–	–	–
Sweden	–	4	4
Switzerland	45	252	297
Syria	8	48	56
Thailand	140	391	531
Turkey	8	107	125
Union of Soviet Socialist Republics	–	3	3
Uruguay	2	8	10
Venezuela	5	37	42
Wales	2	5	7
West Indies	1	15	16
Yugoslavia	14	73	87
Total	**2,600**	**11,109**	**13,709**

Source: *JAMA, 202* (1967), 785. Used by permission of the *Journal of the American Medical Association.*

TABLE B10. Number of internships, by medical school affiliation and bed capacity, 1966-1967

Classification	Number of hospitals	Number of approved programs	Number of internships				Foreign graduates		Total internship positions offered 1968-1969
			Total positions offered Sept. 1, 1966	Total positions filled Sept. 1, 1966	Positions vacant Sept. 1, 1966	Percent filled	Number on duty Sept. 1, 1966	Percent in filled positions	
Nonaffiliated									
Combined Hospitals	15	55	269	169	100	63	76	45	287
Less Than 200 Beds	37	43	253	164	89	65	134	82	280
200-299	129	260	1,226	802	424	65	542	68	1,263
300-499	208	556	2,592	1,660	932	64	867	52	2,669
500-over	73	222	1,614	1,278	336	79	327	26	1,681
Total	462	1,136	5,954	4,073	1,881	68	1,946	48	6,180
Affiliated									
Combined Hospitals	13	53	508	442	66	87	12	3	640
Less Than 200 Beds	19	45	139	88	51	63	11	9	147
200-299	57	117	663	463	200	70	107	23	718
300-499	127	452	2,189	1,767	422	81	403	23	2,329
500-over	138	575	4,116	3,533	583	86	314	9	4,495
Total	354	1,242	7,615	6,293	1,322	83	847	13	8,329
Grand Total	816	2,378	13,569	10,366	3,203	76	2,793	27	14,509

Source: JAMA, 202 (1967), 766. Used by permission of the Journal of the American Medical Association.

Table B11. Number of residencies, by specialty, in affiliated and nonaffiliated hospitals, 1966-1967

Specialty	Number of approved programs	Total offered Sept. 1, 1966	Filled by non-foreign graduates Sept. 1, 1966	Filled by foreign graduates Sept. 1, 1966	Total filled Sept. 1, 1966	Positions vacant Sept. 1, 1966	% of positions filled	Percent foreign graduates in filled positions	Total positions offered 1968-1969
Affiliated									
Anesthesiology	132	1,235	455	415	870	365	70	43	1,323
Colon and rectal surgery	5	10	3	6	9	1	90	67	9
Dermatology	69	400	322	40	362	38	90	11	428
General practice	25	117	31	8	39	78	33	21	123
Internal medicine	255	4,324	2,900	880	3,780	544	87	23	4,953
Neurological surgery	69	369	302	51	353	16	96	14	368
Neurology	77	543	315	109	424	119	78	26	572
Obstetrics and Gynecology	205	1,829	1,246	382	1,628	201	89	24	1,908
Ophthalmology	116	852	760	61	821	31	96	7	892
Orthopedic surgery	166	1,109	924	116	1,040	69	94	11	1,192
Otolaryngology	78	549	446	49	497	52	91	10	607
Pathology	307	2,016	891	462	1,353	663	67	34	2,170
Pediatrics	162	1,750	1,007	498	1,505	245	86	33	1,963
Pediatric allergy	33	53	21	9	30	23	57	30	64
Pediatric cardiology	45	95	27	33	60	35	63	55	131
Physical medicine	59	318	100	81	181	137	57	45	360
Plastic surgery	43	140	117	17	134	6	96	13	156

		Total appointments (all years)						

Table B11 - continued

Specialty	Number of approved programs	Total offered Sept. 1, 1966	Filled by non-foreign graduates Sept. 1, 1966	Filled by foreign graduates Sept. 1, 1966	Total filled Sept. 1, 1966	Positions vacant Sept. 1, 1966	% of positions filled	Percent foreign graduates in filled positions	Total positions offered 1968-1969
Affiliated									
Psychiatry	141	2,596	1,787	380	2,167	429	84	18	2,904
Child-psychiatry	65	350	206	46	252	98	72	18	405
Radiology	161	1,527	1,057	211	1,268	259	83	17	1,711
Surgery	290	3,840	2,622	880	3,502	338	91	25	4,122
Thoracic-surgery	65	182	101	66	167	15	92	40	184
Urology	132	650	461	111	572	78	88	19	663
Total	2,700	24,854	16,103	4,911	21,014	3,840	85	23	27,208
Nonaffiliated									
Anesthesiology	68	417	120	170	290	127	70	59	487
Colon and rectal surgery	7	13	3	6	9	4	69	67	16
Dermatology	16	101	89	9	98	3	97	9	108
General practice	121	707	101	255	356	351	50	72	712
Internal medicine	195	2,225	960	791	1,751	474	79	45	3,152
Neurological surgery	24	159	106	30	136	23	86	22	174
Neurology	21	159	80	37	117	42	74	32	177
Obsterics and gynecology	186	1,000	512	367	879	121	88	42	1,030
Ophthalmology	52	327	269	45	314	13	96	14	351

Table B11 - continued

Specialty	Number of approved programs	Total offered Sept. 1, 1966	Total appointments (all years)						Total positions offered 1968-1969
			Filled by non-foreign graduates Sept. 1, 1966	Filled by foreign graduates Sept. 1, 1966	Total filled Sept. 1, 1966	Positions vacant Sept. 1, 1966	% of positions filled	Percent foreign graduates in filled positions	
Nonaffiliated									
Orthopedic surgery	101	616	471	99	570	46	93	17	657
Otolaryngology	28	263	197	36	233	30	89	16	273
Pathology	366	1,415	315	402	717	698	51	56	1,470
Pediatrics	127	680	248	317	565	115	83	56	726
Pediatric allergy	5	7	4	2	6	1	86	33	7
Pediatric cardiology	4	12	7	4	11	1	92	36	10
Physical medicine	17	81	21	12	33	48	41	36	91
Plastic surgery	27	67	41	14	55	12	82	26	76
Psychiatry	117	1,897	806	574	1,380	517	73	42	2,033
Child-psychiatry	46	203	86	37	123	80	61	30	222
Radiology	105	628	349	100	449	179	72	22	697
Surgery	331	2,681	1,194	1,146	2,340	341	87	49	2,821
Thoracic surgery	30	99	61	34	95	4	96	36	100
Urology	70	284	106	85	251	33	88	34	291
Total	2,064	14,041	6,206	4,572	10,778	3,263	77	42	15,681
Grand Total	4,764	38,895	22,309	9,483	31,792	7,103	82	30	42,889

Source: *JAMA, 202* (1967), 771. Used by permission of the *Journal of the American Medical Association.*

Table B12. Source of professional income for all active physicians in the United States, December 31, 1966

Source of income	Total active	FMGs	Percent of total active who are FMGs
Group medical practice	28,880	1,719	5.9
Fee for service only, individual practice	120,643	11,251	9.3
Fee for service only, other group or partnership practice	14,009	766	5.5
Fee for service and part-time salary, individual practice	15,968	2,097	13.1
Fee for service and part-time salary, other group or partnership practice	2,147	230	10.7
Full-time salary, but some fee for service, individual practice	7,247	1,099	15.2
Full-time salary, but some fee for service, other group or partnership practice	1,848	231	12.5
Full-time salary only	89,573	22,634	25.3
Total	280,315	40,027	14.3

Source: AMA Physician Records, December 31, 1966

Table B13. Details of professional activities for all physicians in the United States, December 31, 1966

Professional activity	Total active	FMGs	Percent of total active who are FMGs
Full-time general practice or other full-time specialty practice	165,245	14,189	8.5
General practice with some specialty practice	20,602	2,298	11.2
Internship in hospital service	10,153	2,591	25.5
Residency or fellowship in hospital service	34,405	10,971	31.9
Other full-time staff in hospital service	31,246	7,117	22.8
Full-time medical school faculty	10,385	1,446	13.9
Administrative medicine	3,928	271	6.9
Research	4,351	1,144	26.3
Total	280,315	40,027	14.3

Source: AMA Physician Records, December 31, 1966

Table B14. Numbers of licenciates representing new additions to the medical profession, in 10 selected states, 1966

State	Total licenciates	Total FMG licenciates	Percent of total licenciates who are FMGs
Maine	51	45	88
New Hampshire	30	20	67
Rhode Island	16	9	56
North Dakota	13	7	54
Vermont	89	43	48
New Jersey	136	57	42
District of Columbia	91	32	35
Maryland	368	130	35
Delaware	13	4	31
Virginia	250	73	29

Source: *JAMA, 200* (1967), 1071. Used by permission of the *Journal of the American Medical Association.*

Table B15.

a. Performance of all candidates examined by state medical boards, 1966

Country of training	Number of candidates	Number passed	Percent failed
U. S. (84)[a]	4,485	4,296	4.2
Foreign (298)	3,691	2,281	38.2

Source: *JAMA, 200,* (1967), 1055-1117.

[a]Figures in parentheses show number of medical schools.

b. Sample of FMGs' State Board performance, 5 selected years

Year Examined	Number of FMG candidates	Percent failed
1950	799	55.0
1955	1,771	41.4
1960	2,864	29.7
1965	3,011	32.1
1966	3,691	38.2[a]

Source: *JAMA, 200* (1967), 1071. Used by permission of the *Journal of the American Medical Association.*

[a]Highest failure rate for U.S. graduates, 1960-1966, 4.2 percent.

Table B16. Additions to medical profession representing graduates
of foreign medical schools, 1950 - 1966

Year	Number passing examination	Number granted reciprocity and endorsement	Totals	Selected percent of total
1950	267	41	308	5.1
1951	425	25	450	
1952	545	24	569	
1953	662	23	685	
1954	749	23	772	
1955	881	26	907	11.7
1956	34	18	852	
1957	991	23	1,014	
1958	1,129	37	1,166	
1959	1,605	21	1,626	
1960	1,383	36	1,419	17.7
1961	1,557	23	1,580	
1962	1,333	24	1,357	
1963	1,409	42	1,451	
1964	1,239	67	1,306	
1965	1,468[a]	60[b]	1,488	16.6
1966	1,352	58	1,410	
Total:	17,829	571	18,400	16.5

Source: *JAMA, 200* (1967), 1072. Used by permission of the *Journal of
the American Medical Association.*

[a] 35 additional licenses added to last year's figure because 3 boards were
late with reports: Calif. (10); Mass. (20); Virgin Islands (5)

[b] 5 additional licenses added to last year's figures for Guam, which was late
in reporting.

Table B17. Performance of FMGs on State Boards in 13 states, 1966

State	Number examined	Number passed	Failed Number	Failed Percent
California	125	108	17	13.6
Connecticut	89	48	41	46.1
District of Columbia	94	69	25	26.6
Illinois	363	96	267	73.6
Indiana	124	83	41	33.1
Maine	101	58	43	42.6
Maryland	268	175	93	34.7
Michigan	126	126	0	0
New Jersey	135	88	47	34.8
New York	873	426	447	51.2
Pennsylvania	191	172	19	9.9
Texas	93	81	12	12.9
Virginia	456	228	228	50.0

Source: *JAMA, 200* (1967),1071. Used by permission of the *Journal of the American Medical Association.*

Table B18. Nine foreign medical schools from which more than 75 candidates for medical licensure came in 1966, with results of examinations

School	Number examined	Number passed	Failed	
			Number	Percent
Universidad Nacional de Buenos Aires	82	56	26	31.7
Universidad de la Habana Cuba	400	231	169	42.0
Universidad de la Santo Domingo	111	45	66	59.5
University of Teheran	111	75	36	32.4
Università degli Studi di Bologna, Facolta di Medicina	92	48	44	47.8
Universidad Nacional Autonoma de Mexico	87	52	35	40.2
University of Santo Tomas, Manila	280	170	110	39.3
Manila Central University	91	43	48	52.7
Istanbul University, Turkey	158	73	85	53.8

Source: *JAMA, 200* (1967), 1071. Used by permission of the *Journal of the American Medical Association.*

Table B19. Numbers of foreign-trained physicians licensed by state boards, 1946-1966

State	Reciprocity and endorsement										Grand totals
	1946-1958	1959	1960	1961	1962	1963	1964	1965	1966	Totals	
Alabama	4	2	0	0	1	0	0	0	0	7	26
Alaska	0	0	1	0	1	0	0	1	0	3	12
Arizona	10	0	0	0	0	0	0	0	0	10	120
Arkansas	2	0	0	0	0	0	0	0	0	2	3
California	50	0	0	0	0	0	0	0	2	52	1,623
Colorado	0	0	1	0	0	0	0	1	0	2	110
Connecticut	159	4	0	1	2	0	0	0	1	167	1,376
Delaware	11	0	4	4	8	9	13	3	11	63	110
District of Columbia	136	32	32	36	41	30	34	23	24	388	745
Florida	0	0	0	0	0	0	0	0	0	0	508
Georgia	22	8	11	10	16	15	10	10	16	118	281
Hawaii	0	0	0	0	0	0	0	0	0	0	67
Idaho	0	0	0	0	0	0	0	0	0	0	9
Illinois	3	0	0	1	0	2	3	11	5	25	2,492
Indiana	74	28	20	3	9	18	0	2	19	173	458
Iowa	38	9	8	7	9	18	15	8	17	129	223
Kansas	0	0	0	0	0	0	0	0	0	0	96
Kentucky	4	1	1	1	3	1	0	0	0	11	129
Louisiana	0	0	0	0	0	0	0	0	0	0	15
Maine	42	10	15	29	16	1	2	3	10	128	733
Maryland	9	0	0	0	0	0	1	0	0	10	1,270
Massachusetts	19	0	0	1	1	0	1	0	0	22	458
Michigan	86	13	16	20	20	33	42	40	49	319	1,094
Minnesota	1	0	0	0	0	0	0	0	5	6	280
Mississippi	2	0	0	0	0	1	0	0	0	3	83
Missouri	8	0	0	0	0	0	0	0	1	9	269
Montana	3	1	3	0	3	2	4	2	0	18	34

Table B19 - continued

State	Reciprocity and endorsement - continued										Grand totals
	1946-1958	1959	1960	1961	1962	1963	1964	1965	1966	Totals	
Nebraska	12	1	1	1	0	0	5	3	1	24	39
Nevada	1	0	0	0	0	0	0	0	0	1	2
New Hampshire	48	5	9	7	5	19	24	23	35	175	295
New Jersey	343	22	21	14	2	2	0	1	0	405	1,555
New Mexico	20	0	1	1	0	0	0	1	2	25	69
New York	271	5	12	7	15	25	94	240	296	965	6,342
North Carolina	11	2	0	0	0	0	0	0	1	14	94
North Dakota	0	0	1	0	1	0	0	0	0	2	95
Ohio	400	94	116	134	122	130	159	130	168	1,453	2,739
Oklahoma	6	2	2	0	3	2	0	1	0	16	19
Oregon	0	0	0	0	0	0	0	0	0	0	52
Pennsylvania	0	0	0	0	0	0	0	0	0	0	1,310
Rhode Island	21	0	1	7	3	11	6	11	13	73	483
South Carolina	0	0	0	0	0	0	0	0	0	0	25
South Dakota	5	2	2	3	1	0	4	2	1	20	105
Tennessee	11	5	11	7	8	7	7	7	10	73	87
Texas	39	7	3	12	25	18	31	29	46	210	925
Vermont	14	0	4	1	10	8	13	21	31	102	187
Virginia	16	0	0	1	0	0	0	1	1	19	1,926
Washington	52	24	26	13	22	18	16	14	9	194	456
West Virginia	0	0	0	0	0	0	0	0	0	0	114
Wisconsin	39	12	22	20	26	15	9	17	18	178	411
Wyoming	2	0	0	1	1	0	9	2	2	17	19
Territories and possessions	39	0	4	3	4	6	18	9	11	94	932
Total	2,033	289	348	372	369	373	520	616	805	5,725	30,905

Source: *JAMA*, 200 (1967), 1107. Used by permission of the *Journal of the American Medial Association*.

APPENDIX B

Table B19. Numbers of foreign-trained physicians licensed by state boards, 1946-1966

State	1946-1958	Examination 1959	1960	1961	1962	1963	1964	1965	1966	Totals
Alabama	11	0	2	0	0	1	4	1	0	19
Alaska	1	0	1	0	1	1	3	2	0	9
Arizona	16	7	13	16	14	15	15	10	4	110
Arkansas	1	0	0	0	0	0	0	0	0	1
California	919	85	97	98	42	57	93	72	108	1,571
Colorado	49	2	3	4	6	13	7	16	8	108
Connecticut	342	136	157	136	84	92	99	115	48	1,209
Delaware	16	1	3	3	5	5	2	6	6	47
District of Columbia	60	14	6	9	35	33	78	53	69	357
Florida	156	32	32	41	45	41	53	77	31	508
Georgia	45	19	9	9	8	12	21	24	16	163
Hawaii	0	9	5	6	9	8	8	11	11	67
Idaho	1	0	0	0	0	4	1	2	1	9
Illinois	1,335	345	132	82	144	123	96	114	96	2,467
Indiana	42	15	25	13	32	18	34	23	83	285
Iowa	47	1	10	9	4	5	10	4	4	94
Kansas	17	9	7	6	6	21	11	12	7	96
Kentucky	1	0	0	0	23	17	27	7	43	118
Louisiana	6	0	0	0	0	0	0	0	9	15
Maine	163	19	35	73	95	75	42	45	58	605
Maryland	544	51	56	72	51	87	109	115	175	1,260
Massachusetts	137	42	37	31	31	40	32	39	47	436
Michigan	180	33	47	66	58	68	100	97	126	775
Minnesota	131	10	13	24	14	15	21	20	26	274
Mississippi	17	3	9	21	12	4	5	6	3	80
Missouri	79	36	1	18	25	17	15	32	37	260
Montana	1	1	0	1	3	8	1	1	0	16

Table B19 - continued

State		Examination - continued								
	1946-1958	1959	1960	1961	1962	1963	1964	1965	1966	Totals
Nebraska	6	3	2	2	2	0	0	0	0	15
Nevada	1	0	0	0	0	0	0	0	0	1
New Hampshire	27	2	2	8	18	10	7	22	24	120
New Jersey	321	136	107	85	106	98	107	102	88	1,150
New Mexico	14	2	4	5	3	7	3	1	5	44
New York	2,113	343	509	350	345	307	593	391	426	5,377
North Carolina	32	2	7	4	1	8	1	9	16	80
North Dakota	40	3	0	6	15	1	1	9	18	93
Ohio	742	90	109	72	56	53	66	58	40	1,286
Oklahoma	2	0	0	0	0	0	0	1	0	3
Oregon	2	1	5	8	10	7	9	2	8	52
Pennsylvania	120	72	85	131	203	170	156	201	172	1,310
Rhode Island	255	25	22	18	27	15	12	25	11	410
South Carolina	1	0	2	5	5	5	6	0	1	25
South Dakota	39	7	6	5	8	6	9	1	4	85
Tennessee	9	1	2	1	0	1	0	0	0	14
Texas	166	40	53	44	63	94	108	66	81	715
Vermont	1	0	2	1	7	10	7	16	41	85
Virginia	386	122	253	237	229	156	140	156	228	1,907
Washington	59	18	29	25	19	16	22	36	38	262
West Virginia	29	4	7	9	13	14	15	8	15	114
Wisconsin	34	13	14	22	20	18	29	37	46	233
Wyoming	1	0	0	0	1	0	0	0	0	2
Territories and possessions	300	116	93	114	82	85	37	8	3	838
Totals	9,017	1,870	2,013	1,890	1,980	1,861	2,215	2,053	2,281	25,180

Table B20. Requirements for medical licensure for physicians trained outside of U.S. and Canada, 1966

State	Citizenship	Internship[a]	ECFMG Certification	Additional Requirements
Alabama	Yes	Yes	Yes	Yes
Alaska	Yes	Yes	No	No
Arizona	Yes	Yes	Yes	Yes
Arkansas	FMGs not accepted			
California	No	Yes	No	Yes
Canal Zone	No	Yes	Yes	Yes
Colorado	Yes	Yes	No	Yes
Connecticut	Declaration of intent	No	No	Yes
Delaware	Yes	Yes	Yes	No
District of Columbia	No	No	Yes	Yes
Florida	Yes	Yes	Yes	Yes
Georgia	Yes	Yes	Yes	No
Guam	No	Yes	Yes	Yes
Hawaii	Declaration of intent	Yes	Yes	Yes
Idaho	Declaration of intent	Yes	Yes	Yes
Illinois	No	No	No	Yes
Indiana	Declaration of intent	Yes	No	Yes
Iowa	Declaration of intent	Yes	Yes	Yes
Kansas	Yes	Yes	No	Yes
Kentucky	Yes	Yes	Yes	Yes
Louisiana	FMGs not accepted			
Maine	No	Yes	Yes	Yes
Maryland	Declaration of intent	Yes	Yes	Yes
Massachusetts	Declaration of intent	No	Yes	Yes
Michigan	Declaration of intent	Yes	Yes	Yes
Minnesota	Declaration of intent	Yes	Yes	Yes
Mississippi	Yes	No	Yes	Yes

Table B20 - continued

State	Citizenship	Internship[a]	ECFMG Certification	Additional Requirements
Missouri	Yes	Yes	Yes	No
Montana	Yes	Yes	Yes	No
Nebraska	Yes	No	Yes	No
Nevada	FMGs not accepted			
New Hampshire	Declaration of intent	Yes	Yes	Yes
New Jersey	Yes	Yes	No	Yes
New Mexico	Declaration of intent	No	Yes	No
New York	Declaration of intent	Yes	Yes	Yes
North Carolina	Yes	No	Yes	Yes
North Dakota	Declaration of intent	Yes	Yes	Yes
Ohio	Yes	Yes	Yes	Yes
Oklahoma	Yes	Yes	Yes	No
Oregon	Declaration of intent	Yes	Yes	Yes
Pennsylvania	Declaration of intent	Yes	Yes	Yes
Puerto Rico	Yes	Yes	No	No
Rhode Island	Declaration of intent	Yes	Yes	Yes
South Carolina	Yes	Yes	Yes	Yes
South Dakota	Declaration of intent	Yes	Yes	Yes
Tennessee	Yes	No	Yes	Yes
Utah	No	Yes	Yes	Yes
Vermont	Declaration of intent	No	Yes	Yes
Virgin Islands	No	Yes	No	No
Virginia	Declaration of intent	Yes	Yes	Yes
Washington	No	Yes	Yes	No
West Virginia	Yes	Yes	Yes	Yes
Wisconsin	Declaration of intent	Yes	Yes	Yes
Wyoming	Yes	Yes	Yes	No

Source: *JAMA*, 200 (1967), 1106. Used by permission of the *Journal of the American Medical Association*.

[a] ECFMG certification is a prerequisite for admission into an approved internship or residency program.

Table B21. Comparison of numbers of FMGs and USMGs who repeated licensure examinations (licensed in 1966)

Total Repeaters	Total USMGs[a]	Total FMGs	% FMGs	FMG 1 previous failure	FMG 2 previous failures	FMG 3 previous failures	FMG 4 previous failures	FMG 5 or more previous failures[b]
456	43	413	91	213	83	39	26	27

Source: *JAMA, 200* (1967), 1060. Used by permission of the *Journal of the American Medical Association.*

[a]Includes three Canadians

[b]The most previous failures by any candidate was 12. The candidate with the second largest numbers of failures was 10. He had taken his examinations in three other states before passing the New York board in 1966.

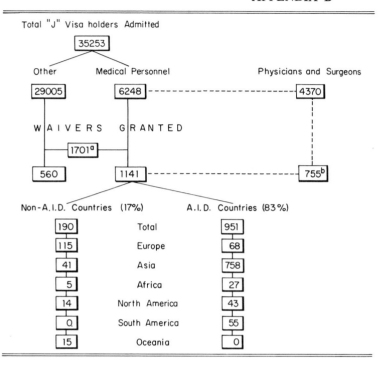

CHART B1. "J" Visa Adjustments: Medical Personnel, Fiscal Year 1966

Source: *The International Migration of Talent and Skills,* Department of State, October 1966.

[a] Figure shown is approximations based on data compiled from the Department of State, Bureau of Educational and Cultural Affairs sources. The actual number of waivers granted, fiscal year 1966, was 1930. (Source: INS)

[b] No breakdown by country is available for physicians and surgeons who obtained waivers, fiscal year 1966.

153

NOTES

NOTES TO PREFACE

1. For a complete discussion of this point, see the AAMC's report to the Agency for International Development: *A World Program for Health Manpower*, Association of American Medical Colleges, Evanston, Ill.: October, 1965.

2. For a comprehensive discussion of foreign research trainees in sponsored programs, a good source is Kelly M. West, "Training for Medical Research: The World Role of the United States," *J. Med. Educ., 39* (No. 3, March 1964), 237–264.

3. Frankel, Charles, "Migration of Talent and Skills, Country Needs and the United States Immigration Act," "Statement Before the Senate Judiciary Committee on Immigration and Naturalization," March 6, 1967, p. 1.

4. "Brain Drain has saved the United States 357 Million," *Home News*, London, December 12, 1966, p. 7. "Medical Brain Drain A Tragic Loss for Korea," *Korean Times*, Seoul, February 4, 1967, p. 3; "Some Reflections on Developing Health Services," a speech by the Minister of Health of Israel, Yissrael Barzilai, Fourth Rehovoth Conference, August 18, 1967, p. 5. Unpublished paper.

5. An excellent reference on the socioeconomic factors involved in migration is *The Determinants and Consequences of Population Trends,* United Nations Document, Population Studies, No. 1, New York: 1953.

6. *Some Facts and Figures on the Migration of Talent and Skills,* prepared by the Staff of the Council on International Education and Cultural Affairs, United States Department of State, Charles Frankel, Assistant Secretary of the Bureau of Educational and Cultural Affairs, Chairman. Washington: February 1967.

NOTES TO CHAPTER I

1. AMA data *Reports.* A special study of the AMA physician tapes done for the National Advisory Commission on Health Manpower, May 19, 1967. Unpublished series of 50 tables of data.

2. *Ibid.*

3. *National Distribution of Physicians, Hospitals, and Hospital Beds*

in the U.S.: Vol. 1, *Metropolitan Areas*. Chicago: AMA, 1966, pp. 143–170.

4. This particular information function is not the responsibility of the INS, however. One of the most informative sources of information on United States citizens who have received their medical education abroad is David McLean Greeley's "American Foreign Medical Graduates," *J. Med. Educ., 41* (1966), 641–650.

5. "Medical Education in the United States, 1965–1966," *JAMA* 198 (1966), 874–938.

6. Visa data available in the tables of *Some Facts and Figures on the Migration of Talent and Skills*, Bureau of Educational and Cultural Affairs, State Department, May, 1967.

7. All of these data pertaining to FMGs in internships and residencies are available in "Medical Education in the United States, 1965–1966."

8. "Foreign Physicians, Many Unqualified, Fill Vacuum in the United States," *New York Times*, September 29, 1967, pp. 1, 31. Quoted from a statement made to the N.Y. Times reporter, Richard D. Lyons, by Peter Olim, Director of the Korea Travel Service in New York City.

9. *National Distribution of Physicians, Hospitals, and Hospital Beds in the United States*, Vol. 2, pp. 320–331.

10. Section 266 (b) of the Immigration and Nationality Act states that: "Any alien or any parent or legal guardian in the United States of any alien who fails to give written notice to the Attorney General, as required by Section 265 of this title, shall be guilty of a misdemeanor and shall, upon conviction thereof, be fined not to exceed $200 or be imprisoned not more than 30 days, or both. Irrespective of whether an alien is convicted and punished as herein provided, any alien who fails to give written notice to the Attorney General, as required by Section 265, shall be taken into custody in the manner provided by Chapter 5 of this title, unless such alien established to the satisfaction of the Attorney General that such failure was reasonably excusable or was not willful."

11. AMA *Proceedings* of the House of Delegates, Atlantic City: June 18–22, 1967, pp. 55–56.

12. "Employment Service Review," Bureau of Employment Security, U.S. Department of Labor, *3* (1966), 8.

13. "Indicators," U.S. Department of Health, Education and Welfare, January, 1967, p. 5.

14. Report of the National Advisory Commission on Health Manpower, *1* (1967), 13–15.

15. "Medicine, Money, and Manpower: The Challenge to Professional Education," *New Engl. J. Med. 276* (1967), 1414–1422.

16. Rashi Fein, *The Doctor Shortage*, Washington: Brookings Institution, May, 1967, pp. 79–89, 134–140.

17. "Medical Education in the United States," p. 891.

NOTES TO CHAPTER II

1. David McLean Greeley, "American Foreign Medical Graduates," *J. Med. Educ., 41* (1966), 641–650.

2. *JAMA*, State Board Number *192* (1967), 853–904.

3. *Annual Report*, ECFMG, 1963, p. 22.

4. G. Halsey Hunt, "Some Problems of the ECFMG," a speech presented at the Annual Examination Institute, The Federation of State Medical Boards of the United States, Chicago, February 5, 1966.

5. ECFMG, *Annual Report*, 1963, p. 22.

6. *JAMA*, State Board Issue, *200* (1967), 198–199.

7. *Ibid.*, p. 1070.

NOTES TO CHAPTER III

1. *World Directory of Medical Schools*, World Health Organization, Geneva, 1963.

2. Harold Margulies, Lucille S. Bloch, and Francis K. Cholko, "Random Survey of U.S. Hospitals with Approved Internships and Residencies: A Study of the Professional Qualities of FMGs," *J. Med. Educ., 43* (1968), 706–716.

3. *Ibid.* Hospital Administrators in 28 hospitals listed 1 foreign medical school as having sent them their best FMGs, while administrators in another 18 hospitals listed that same medical school as the one which had sent them their worst FMGs.

4. Jacob C. Halberstam and Michael M. Dacso, "Foreign and U.S. Residents in University-Affiliated Hospitals: An Investigation of U.S. Graduate Medical Education," *Bull. N.Y. Acad. Med., Second Series, 42* (1966), 182–208.

5. *JAMA*, State Board Issue, *200* (1967), 1055–1120.

6. *Ibid.*, pp. 1055–1120. All of these data are contained in the State Board issue of the *JAMA*. Those given in this monograph represent the more salient points in state licensure experience with FMGs, although they constitute only a minor portion of the valuable data brought together each year in the State Board issues.

7. This number (30,000) includes American citizens who have been trained abroad.

NOTES TO CHAPTER IV

1. Tycho Brahe, quoted in *Brain Drain and Brain Gain: A Bibliography on Migration of Scientists, Engineers, Doctors, and Students*, published by the Research Policy Program, Lund, Sweden: 1967, p. 1.

2. Mary McGrath, *Boston Herald.*

3. U.S. Department of State, Bureau of Security and Consular Affairs Circular, October 25, 1965.

4. *Federal Register*, Codified document, Schedules A & B, December 3, 1965, p. 14979.

5. "The Council's Concern with the Brain Drain," A Progress Report from the Bureau of Cultural Affairs, U.S. Department of State, March 18, 1966. "Educational and Cultural Exchange: Failure of Academic Visitors to Return Home After Completing Their Programs in the United States," Bureau of Cultural Affairs Circular, August 11, 1966.

6. Herbert G. Grubel, "The Brain Drain: A U.S. Dilemma," *Science, 154* (1966), 1420-1423; Peter Kayser, *Reuters*, the "Brain Drain Conference," Lausanne: August 25, 1967, p. 8.

7. "Some Facts and Figures on the Migration of Talent and Skills," Council of International Education and Cultural Affairs, May, 1967.

8. The 1-94 file on every alien would be an ideal method for recording departures from the United States, since every alien is supposed to surrender his 1-94 card when he leaves the country. To date, however, the INS has not followed through and recorded departures in any systematic manner that is available for public scrutiny.

9. "The Brain Drain into the U.S. of Scientists, Engineers, and Physicians," A Staff Study for the Research and Technical Programs Subcommittee of the Committee on Government Operations, Henry S. Reuss, Chairman, July 1967, p. 3.

10. This point should be emphasized, for there are some who contend that the McCarran-Walter Act of 1952 also stressed skills, since it permitted 50 percent of the visas given to persons eligible under the First Preference category to be granted to professional or skilled persons. Under that arrangement, however, the national origins quota remained in effect, thereby favoring the more advanced nations.

11. Reuss Subcommittee Report, p. 4.

12. "Migration of Talent and Skills," pp. 65-90.

13. "Medical School Expenditures for Regular Operating Programs," AAMC *Datagrams, 8* (1967).

14. Data compiled from INS and AAMC statistics.

NOTES TO CHAPTER V

1. Quote from an anonymous British immigrant to America, in "Migration from Developed Countries: The Case of Britain," an unpublished preliminary draft of the Advisory Committee on Medical Research, Pan American Health Organization, Washington, D.C., p. 31.

2. *AMA News, 10* (1967), 8.

3. Francisco T. Dalupan, "Critical Aspects of Philippines Education," University of the East, Department of University Publications, Manila, April, 1964.

4. The New York Times reported that the shortage of physicians in the United States is reaching "alarming proportions" (June 19, 1967) and that foreign interns and residents in United States hospitals are there "largely because without them American medical services would go into a tailspin" (December 18, 1966, p. E 11).

5. Richard M. Titmuss, "Welfare State and Welfare Society," address before the Sixth British National Conference on Social Welfare, April 10, 1966.

6. *Parliamentary Debates*, House of Lords Official Report, Lord Windlesham's speech on the Brain Drain, Tuesday, December 20, 1966; Peter Kayser, *Reuters Press*, Lausanne, August 25, 1967; Louis Parai, "Immigration and Emigration of Professional and Skilled Manpower During the Postwar Period," Special Study Number 1, prepared for the Economic Council of Canada, Ottawa, June, 1965.

NOTES TO CHAPTER VI

1. E. M. Friedwald, "The Research Effort of Western Europe, the U.S.A. and the U.S.S.R.," OECD *Observer*, Special Issue on Science, February, 1966.

2. "Wilson Censure Defeated," *The Washington Post*, February 14, 1967, p. A 14.

3. "Brain Drain Curbs by U.S. is Opposed," *The New York Times*, March 6, 1967, p. 23.

4. "Migration of Health Personnel, Scientists, and Engineers from Latin America," Pan American Health Organization, 1966.

5. These same criteria could be applied equally to graduates of United States medical schools. We have avoided dealing with that issue, for the focus of this monograph is on FMGs, not USMGs. A separate study might very well prove that USMGs require the same reevaluative procedures as those described for FMGs.

NOTES TO APPENDIX A

1. The Chairman of this Committee was Dr. Donald Anderson, Dean of the School of Medicine and Dentistry of the University of Rochester. The Secretary of the Cooperating Committee was Dr. Walter S. Wiggins, then Associate Secretary of the Council on Medical Education and Hospitals of the AMA. *Annual Report of the ECFMG*, 1958, p. 4.

2. *Annual Report*, ECFMG, 1958, p. 4.

3. G. Halsey Hunt, "Some Problems of the ECFMG," a speech

presented at the Annual Examination Institute, The Federation of State Medical Boards of the United States, Palmer House, Chicago, February 5, 1966, p. 2.

4. *Ibid.*, pp. 6–7.

5. Proceedings of House of Delegates, American Hospital Association, August 18, 19, and 20, 1958, p. 38.

6. *Annual Report*, ECFMG, 1963, p. 22.

BIBLIOGRAPHY

ARTICLES, SPEECHES, AND JOURNALS

Fox, Melvin J., "Some Pluses and Minuses of the So-Called Brain Drain," presented at the 8th World Conference of the Society for International Development, 1966.

Friedwald, E. M., "The Research Effort of Western Europe, the USA, and the USSR," *OECD Observer*, special issue on Science, Feb. 1966.

Grubel, Herbert G., "Nonreturning Foreign Students and the Cost of Student Exchange." *International Educational and Cultural Exchange*, a publication of the U.S. Advisory Commission on International Educational and Cultural Affairs. Spring 1966, pp. 20–29.

Grubel, Herbert G., "The Brain Drain: A U.S. Dilemma," *Science, 154*, (December 16, 1966), 1420–1423.

Grubel, Herbert G., and A. D. Scott, "The International Flow of Human Capital," *American Economic Review, 56* (No. 2, May 1966), 268–274.

Halberstam, Jacob L., and Michael M. Dacso, "Foreign and United States Residents in University Affiliated Teaching Hospitals: An Investigation of United States Graduate Medical Education"; *Bulletin of the New York Academy of Medicine, March 1966.*

Haniotis, George V., "An Exercise in Voluntary Repatriation in Greece," *OECD Observer*, August 1964, pp. 12–15.

Henderson, Gregory, "Foreign Students: Exchange or Immigration?", *Foreign Service Journal, 42* (April 1965), 36–37, 49 (Also available in *International Development Review, 6* [No. 4], 19–21).

Henry, David D., "University Problems in Recruitment of Teaching and Research Personnel from Abroad," *Educational Record, 48* (No. 1, Winter 1967), 51–60.

House of Lords, *Parliamentary Debates*, London, Dec. 20, 1966.

Hunt, G. Halsey, "The Brain Drain in Medicine," *Federation Bulletin* (published monthly by the Federation of State Medical Boards of the United States, Inc., Fulton, Missouri, 65251), *53* (April 1966), 98–107.

Hyde, Henry van Zile, speech before 72nd Annual Meeting of AAMC regarding the ECFMG, *Journal of Medical Education, 37* (No. 3, March 1962), 165–170.

BIBLIOGRAPHY

Kidd, Charles V., "The Growth of Science and the Distribution of Scientists Among the Nations." *Impact of Science on Society, 14* (1964), 5–18.

Miller, Henry, "In Sickness and in Health: A Doctor's View of Medicine in Britain," *Encounter, 28* (No. 4, April 1967), 10–21.

Myers, Robert G., "The 'Brain Drain' and Foreign Student Nonreturn," *Exchange,* Spring 1967, pp. 63–73.

Perkins, J. A., "Foreign Aid and the Brain Drain," *Foreign Affairs, 44* (No. 4, July 1966), 608–619.

The Annals of the American Academy of Political Science, 367 (September 1966).

West, Kelly M., "Training for Medical Research: The World Role of the United States." *J. Med. Educ., 39* (March 1964), 237–264.

West, Kelly M., "Foreign Interns and Residents in U.S.," *J. Med. Educ., 40* (1965), 1110–1129.

Wolfe, Dael, "Brain Drain," [editorial] *Science, 154* (Nov. 25, 1966).

BOOKS

Commager, Henry Steele. *The American Mind.* New Haven and London: Yale University Press, 1950.

Faulkner, H. V. *American Political and Social History.* New York: Appleton-Century-Crofts, Inc., 1952.

Langer, William L. *An Encyclopedia of World History.* Boston: Houghton Mifflin Company, 1957.

Morrison, Samuel Eliot. *The Oxford History of the American People.* New York: Oxford University Press, 1965.

Musgrove, Frank. *The Migratory Elite.* London: Hineman, 1963.

Thomas, Brinley, Ed. *Economics of International Migration.* London: International Economic Association, 1958.

CONGRESSIONAL REFERENCES

Frankel, Charles. "Migration of Talent and Skills, Country Needs and the U.S. Immigration Act," Statement before Senate Judiciary Subcommittee on Immigration and Naturalization, March 6, 1967. Unpublished.

Kidd, Charles V. "Statement on the Migration of Highly Trained Persons"; Before the Senate Judiciary Subcommittee on Immigration and Naturalization, March 6, 1967.

Mondale, Walter F. "The Brain Drain from Developing Countries," *Congressional Record,* 89th Congress, 2nd Session, Vol. 112, September 9, 1966, pp. 21262–21274.

Mondale, Walter F. "The International Brain Drain Act," *Congressional*

BIBLIOGRAPHY

Record, 89th Congress, Vol. 112, No. 176, October 13, 1966, pp. 25438–25446.

Noto, Mario T. Associate Commissioner, Operations, Immigration and Naturalization Service, United States Department of Justice. "Statement before the Immigration and Nationality (Subcommittee #1) House Judiciary Committee April 19, 1967 on Exchange Visitors," unpublished.

Nunemaker, John C., M.D., Director of the Department of Graduate Medical Education of the American Medical Association. "Statement of the American Medical Association, Re: Immigration Aspects of the Mutual Educational and Cultural Exchange Act, before Subcommittee No. 1, Committee on the Judiciary, House of Representatives, April 26, 1967." Unpublished.

Reuss, Henry S. *The Brain Drain Into the U. S. of Scientists, Engineers, and Physicians*, A Staff Study for the Research and Technical Programs, Subcommittee of the House of Representatives, Committee on Government Operations, July, 1967.

Reuss, Henry S. "The Brain Drain of Scientists, Engineers, and Physicians from the Developing Countries into the United States," Hearing before a Subcommittee of the Committee on Government Operations, House of Representatives, January 23, 1968. Washington: United States Government Printing Office, 1968.

Reuss, Henry S., "Scientific Brain Drain from the Developing Countries," Twenty-third Report by the Committee on Government Operations, March 28, 1968, House Report No. 1215, Washington: United States Government Printing Office, 1968.

REPORTS AND MONOGRAPHS

AAMC, *A World Program for Health Manpower*, Report to AID, October 1965.

AAMC, *Datagram*, November 1, 1966.

AAMC, *Directory of Medical Schools*. Evanston, 1965–1966.

AAMC, *Manpower for the World's Health*, Report of the 1966 Institute on International Medical Education, 1967.

AMA, *Distribution of Physicians, Hospitals, and Hospital Beds in the U. S.*, Vol. 1 (Regional, State and County), Vol. 2 (Metropolitan Areas), Chicago, 1967.

Annual Reports, Educational Council for Foreign Medical Graduates, 1958–1965.

"Brain Drain and Brain Gain," Research Policy Program. Lund, Sweden, 1967.

Brihley, Thomas. *International Migration and Economic Development.* UNESCO: Turin, 1961.

BIBLIOGRAPHY

Bulletin on International Education, American Council on Education, Position Paper on "International Migration of Intellectual Talent." Nov. 17, 1966.

Council on International Educational and Cultural Affairs. "The Problem of the Nonreturning Exchange Visitor." Report of the Interagency Task Force of the Council. April 23, 1965. (Available from the Bureau of Educational and Cultural Affairs, Department of State.)

Educational Council for Foreign Medical Graduates, *Handbook for Foreign Medical Graduates*, 1965.

Fein, Rashi. *The Doctor Shortage: An Economic Diagnosis*. Brookings Studies in Social Economics. Washington: Brookings Institution, 1967.

Gutierrez Olivos, Sergio, and Riguelme Perez, Jorge. "La emigracion de recursos humanos de alto nivel y el caso de Chile." Washington, D.C.: Pan American Union, 1965.

Immigration and Naturalization Service. *Annual Report*, 1966.

Institute of International Exchange. "Report on International Exchange," *Open Doors*, New York, 1965.

Millis, John S., *et al*. *The Graduate Education of Physicians*, The Report of the Citizens Commission on Graduate Medical Education to the Council of Medical Education. Chicago: AMA, August 1966.

Naficy, Habib. "The 'Brain Drain': The Case of Iranian Non-returnees." Embassy of Iran, Washington, D.C. (A report presented at the annual Conference of the Society of International Development, New York City, March 17, 1966.)

Pan American Health Organization. *Migration of Health Personnel, Scientists, and Engineers from Latin America*, September 1966.

Royal Society of London. "Emigration of Scientists from the United Kingdom." Report of a Committee Appointed by the Royal Society, 1963.

Scalcione, Peter. *The Impact of the Exchange and Immigrant Medical Graduate on the New York City Municipal Hospital System* (Unpublished thesis for the Baruch School of Business and Public Administration, August, 1966).

United States Advisory Commission on International Educational and Cultural Affairs. "Foreign Students in the United States: A National Survey." 1966. (Available from the Bureau of Educational and Cultural Affairs, Department of State.) Also: "Some Facts and Figures on the Migration of Talent and Skills."

Wilson, James. "Investigation of 765 British Migrant Scientists in the United States and Canada." (Unpublished Ph.D. dissertation, Queens University, Belfast Ireland, 1964; available through the University of Pittsburgh Library.)

World Health Organization. *World Directory of Medical Schools*, Geneva, 1963.

INDEX

Agency for International Development (AID), v, 94

American Hospital Association (AHA): supports FMGs, v; FMG regulatory mechanisms of, 28–29; suggested policy decisions for, 93–97; helps establish Cooperating Committee, 103–104; represented on committee making recommendations to ECFMG, 113–114

American Medical Association (AMA), viii; supports FMGs, v; data on active physicians in United States, 1; data on FMGs, 1–2, 3, 19; on health manpower shortages, 22; Council on Medical Education and Hospitals, 25, 27; Liaison Committee, 26–27; FMG regulatory mechanisms of, 29; on ECFMG *vs.* National Board examinations, 36; controls status of medical schools, 44–45; suggested policy decisions for, 93–97; helps establish Cooperating Committee, 103–104; represented on committee making recommendations to ECFMG, 113–114; "The Quality of Medicine is Strained," 36

American Medical Qualification Examination, 106, 108

American Republican Party, 64

Annual Examination Institute of the Federation of State Medical Boards, 35

Arkansas: absence of FMGs in, 29

Association of American Medical Colleges (AAMC): supports FMGs, v; Liaison Committee, 26–27; Executive Committee, 27; controls status of medical schools, 44–45; sponsors study of FMGs' professional quality, 49–52; suggested policy decisions for, 93–97, 99; helps establish Cooperating Committee, 103–104; represented on committee making recommendations to ECFMG, 113–114

Australia: immigration exclusion policy of, 64

Baltimore: non-patient care physicians in, 15

Brahe, Tycho, 59

Brain drain: concern of India, Canada, Greece, and Israel over, vii–viii; Great Britain's concern over, vii–viii, 78, 83, 88–89; related to socioeconomic development, viii–ix, 85, 88; related to immigration policies, 75, 77; defined, 78; related to health manpower shortages, 79–84, 86; factor of FMGs' graduate training in United States related to his service to home country, 84–85, 86, 89; salary scale factor of, 90. *See also* Health manpower problem

California: requirements for FMGs in, 29

Canada: brain drain in, vii, 83; United States qualifications for

medical graduates from, 2, 29;
FMGs in, 20, 22
Conference on International Education in Medicine, 31, 33, 113
Consultant Group on Medical Education, 23
Convention of Buenos Aires (*1936*), 65
Convention of Caracas (*1954*), 65

Dalupan, Francisco T.: on brain drain, 81
Darley, Ward: on physician shortage, 23
Dacso, Michael M.: on FMGs as hospital trainees, 52
Delaware: requirements for FMGs in, 29
Dominican Republic: FMGs from, 80

Educational Council for Foreign Medical Graduates (ECFMG): India bans examination of, vii, 43; Canadians exempted from examination of, 2, 29; establishment, 25, 103–105; certification requirements, 28–31; growth of examination candidate list, 31–33, 108, 109–112, 115; states primary functions (*1962*), 33–34, 35, 114; major accomplishments, 34; major problems, 35, 40–41; examination of *vs.* National Board examination, 35–36; FMGs' percentage distribution on examination, 35–36, 37–38, 53, 54; conflict between original purpose of examination and present policies, 36, 39–40; relations with Labor Department, 40, 42; relations with State Department, 42; influences immigration laws, 42; criticism of, 42–43; examination requirements, 52–53; purpose of examination, 53; suggested policy decisions for, 93–97; original

functions of, 104; criteria for basic requirements, 105–106; Examination Committee, 106; gives control of examination to National Board, 106; examination policies, 106–107; revises examination, 108; revises educational requirements for examination, 108, 113; Temporary Certificates policy, 113; recommendations of Steering Committee to, 113–114; Board of Trustee membership, 115; *Fact Book*, 6; *Annual Report* for *1962* and for *1965*, 33, 35; *Handbook for Foreign Medical Graduates*, 34
Educational Testing Service, 44, 106
Exchange Visitor Program: evaluated, x, 86; as avenue of immigration, 66–67, 68; waivers granted under, 67, 74. *See also* Exchange Visitor visa
Exchange Visitor visa (J visa): INS data on, 4; *vs.* Permanent Resident visa, 9, 19–20, 66; as used by FMGs, 13, 66; waivers of, 20, 67; classification, 68; granting of, 68–69; Forms DSP/37 and DSP/66, 69; INS Form 1–94, 69; status of FMGs with, 71
Exchange Visitor's Waiver Review Board, 67

Federation of State Medical Boards: helps establish committee on FMGs, 103–104
Fein, Rashi: on future need for health services, 23
Foreign Medical Graduates (FMGs), *passim*; prototypic descriptions of, 4–9; home countries, 9, 74; as hospital trainees, 9–13, 24, 49–52, 84–85, 92; national distribution, 14–19; certification of, 19–20, 21, 26, 28–33 *passim*, 55; definition of, 28;

166

INDEX

Indiana: requirements for FMGs in, 29

Institut de Medicina si Farmacia (Romania), 47

Institute for International Education: *Open Doors*, 9

Iran: FMGs from, 80

Israel: reacts to brain drain, vii–viii

Japan: medical schools in, 46

Journal of the American Medical Association, 53

J visa, see Exchange Visitor visa

Kansas: requirements for FMGs in, 29

Korea, FMGs from, 74

Kosygin, Alexei: on brain drain, 89

Labor Department: reports physician shortage, 22; relations with ECFMG, 40, 42; Labor Certification, 63–64; ruling on Permanent Resident visas for FMGs, 71–72; defines physician, 72

Lebanon: medical schools in, 46

Louisiana: absence of FMGs in, 29

McCarran-Walter Act, see Immigration Act of *1952*

Maine: FMGs in, 19

Marcos, Pacifico: on brain drain, 81

Maryland: licensure requirements for FMGs in, 55

Massachusetts: requirements for FMGs in, 29

Medical schools: FMGs at, viii, ix; respond to physician shortage, 23–24; accrediting procedures, 26–27, 44–45; types of graduates from, 27–28; in foreign countries, 46–49; construction and operating costs, 75

Michigan: FMG failure rate on state examination, 54

Middle Atlantic states: ratio of physicians to population, 3

Mutual Education and Cultural Exchange Act (Fulbright-Hayes Act of *1961*), 66, 67, 68

National Advisory Commission on Health Manpower: reports on physician shortage, 22–23; sponsors survey of FMGs' professional quality, 49–52

National Board of Medical Examiners: National Board *vs.* ECFMG examinations, 35–36; National Board *vs.* State Board examinations, 45, 54–55; quality of examinations of, 95; assumes control of ECFMG examinations, 106

National Intern Matching Plan, 11

Nevada: absence of FMGs in, 29

New England states: ratio of physicians to population, 3

New Hampshire: FMGs in, 19

New Jersey: FMGs in, 11; requirements for FMGs, 29; Hospital Research and Educational Trust, 34

New York, FMGs in, 14; requirements for FMGs, 29–30, 55; failure rates of FMGs on state examination, 55

New York City: ratio of physicians to population, 3; physicians in non-patient care, 14

New York University: Hospital Research and Educational Trust, 34

Nicaragua: FMGs from, 80

North Dakota: FMGs in, 19

Peace Corps, 46–47

Permanent Resident visa: *vs.* Exchange Visitor visa, 9, 19–20, 66; related to liberalization of immigration policy, 61, 64; classification of, 68; preference